Medicine in the M

Extracts from "Le Moye

Edmond Dupouy

(Translator: Thomas C. Minor)

Alpha Editions

This edition published in 2022

ISBN : 9789356895157

Design and Setting By
Alpha Editions
www.alphaedis.com
Email - info@alphaedis.com

Contents

THE PHYSICIANS OF THE MIDDLE AGES.

In the fourth century of the Christian era Roman civilization expired; Western Europe was invaded by the barbarians; letters and science sought a last refuge at Alexandria; the Middle Age commenced.

Greek medicine strove to survive the revolution in the city of the Ptolemies, and even produced a few celebrated physicians, *i.e.*, Alexander Ætius, Alexander Trallian, and Paulus Ægineta, but at the end of the seventh century the school of Alexandria also fell and disappeared in the clouds of a false philosophy, bequeathing all Hippocratic traditions to the Arabs, who advanced as conquerors to the Occident.

The Arabian schools of Dschondisabur, Bagdad, Damascus, and Cordova were founded and became flourishing institutions of learning, thanks to a few Nestorian Greeks and Jews who were attracted to these centers of learning; such men as Aaron, Rhazes, Haly-Abas, Avicenna, Avenzoar, Averrhoes, Albucasis, and other writers, who continued the work left by the Greeks, leaving remarkable books on medicine and surgery. Unfortunately the ordinance of Islamism prevented these scientists from following anatomical work too closely, and consequently limited the progress they might otherwise have made in medicine.[1]

What occurred in Western Europe during this period of transition? The torch of science was extinguished; the sacred fire on the altar of learning only remained a flickering emblem whose pale light was carefully guarded in the chapel of monasteries. Medicine was abandoned to the priests, and all practice naturally fell into an empirical and blind routine. "The physician-clergy," says Sprengel, "resorted in the majority of cases to prayers and holy water, to the invocations of saints and martyrs, and inunction with sacred ointments. These monks were unworthy of the name of doctor—they were, in fact, nothing else than fanatical hospital attendants."

An ephemeral ray of light broke from the clouds in the *renaissance* of 805, when Charlemagne ordered the cathedral schools to add medicine to their studies as a part of the *quadrivium*. Some of the monks now commenced to study the works of Celsus and Cœlius Aurelianus, but, ever as with the Mussulmen, the Catholic religion forbade the dissection of the human body, and the monks made no more progress than the barbarians; so that the masses of the people had little or no confidence in clerical medical skill. We find the proof of a lack of confidence in the Gothic laws promulgated by Theodoric about this period—laws kept even into the eleventh century in the greater portion of Western Europe. These ordinances, among other things, proclaim as follows:

"No physician must open a vein of a woman or a daughter of the nobility without being assisted by a relative or body-servant; *quia difficillium non est, ut sub tali occasione ludibrium interdum adhærescat.*" (Their morality was then a subject for caution.)

"When a physician is called to dress a wound or treat a disease, he must take the precaution to settle on his fee, for he cannot claim any in case the patient's life is endangered.

"He shall be entitled to five sous for operating on hard cataract.

"If a physician wound a gentleman by bleeding, he shall be condemned to pay a fine of one hundred sous; and should the gentleman die following the operation, the physician must be delivered into the hands of the dead man's relatives, who may deal with the doctor as they see fit.

"When a physician has a student he shall be allowed twelve sous for his services as tutor."

Towards the tenth century, however, progress in medicine is at last noticeable. We see some monks going to make their studies at Salerno and at Mount Cassin, where the Benedictine friars had established a medical college in the previous century. Constantine had given these friars Arabian manuscripts, which had been translated into Latin, with commentaries. Also the works of the early Greek physicians and the treatises of Aristotle on "Natural Science." It was at Salerno that Ægidius de Corbeil studied physic before becoming physician to Philip Augustus. Nevertheless, medicine remained in darkness with clerical ignorance, the superstition and despotism of the church offering an insurmountable barrier to all science. Finally a reform was instituted in 1206 by the foundation of the University of Paris, which included among its school of learning a college of medicine, wherein many students matriculated. The *physicus* Hugo, and Obiso, physician to Louis the Great, were the first professors in the institution. Degrees were accorded indiscriminately to the clergy or to the laity, the condition of celibacy being imposed on the latter likewise.

A medical and surgical service was organized at the Hotel Dieu, which hospital was erected before the entrance of Notre Dame, under the direction of the clergy. On certain days the priests would assemble around the holy water font of the cathedral, *supra cupam*, in order to discuss questions in medicine or the connection of scholastic learning with the healing art.

The University only recognized as students of medicine persons who held the degree of master-in-arts. They absolutely separated the *meges* and *mires*, surgeons, bonesetters, and barbers, who had made no classical studies, and to whom was abandoned as unworthy of the real physicians all that concerned minor surgery. These officers of health, so-called, of the Middle

Ages were unimportant and little respected persons; they kept shops and never went out without carrying one or two dressing cases; they were only comparable to drug peddlers; and the University imposed no vows of celibacy in their case.

In many literary works in Latin it is often a question whether to call in a physician or *mire*, and certain passages admirably serve to prove this historical fact. In the *Roman de Dolopatos*,[2] for example, the poet tells how to prevent the poisoning of wounds, as they are easy to cure when the injury is recent:

You have heard it told

To dress a wound while new;

'Tis hard to heal when old.

You'll find this statement true.[3]

When the doctor cometh late

The wound may poisoned be;

The sore may irritate

And most sad results we see.

In another troubadour song, *The Wicked Surgeon* (*Vilain Mire*), from which Moliere purloined his play "A Doctor in Spite of Himself," we see the wife of the bone-setter assure every one that her husband is not only a good surgeon, but likewise knows as much of medicine and uroscopy as Hippocrates himself. (We must not forget that a knowledge of urine was claimed by *mires* and *meges*.) Thus the bone setter's wife says:

"My husband is, as I have said,

A surgeon who can raise the dead.

He sees disease in urine hid,

Knows more than e'en Ypocras did."

The *Roman de la Rose* shows us a poor devil who complains of not being able to find a surgeon (*mire*) to dress his wounds, *i.e.*:

"Ne sceus que faire, ne que dire,

Ne pour ma playe trover mire,

Ne par herbe, ne par racine

Je ne peus trover medecine."

Some years after the founding of the University of Paris, a great scientific movement occurred in the Occident. The Faculty of Montpellier had already acquired much celebrity. The College of Surgeons of Paris was established in 1271. Medical circles counted a brilliant galaxy of remarkable men, *i.e.* Richard de Wendmere, Jean de Saint Amand, Guillaume Saliceto, the great Albert, Bernard Gordon, Arnauld de Villeneuve, Lanfranc, and Roger Bacon. The school of Paris now wished to direct its own affairs, and accordingly, in 1280 A.D., separated from the University and assumed the title *Physicorum Facultas*, and its members became physicians. Sustained by Royal edict, they obtained rich grants from the church and from public taxes, but these marks of favor aroused bitter jealousies; criticism rained down on the healing art on every hand, and medicine was lampooned; these physicians of the thirteenth century were ridiculed so bitterly as to make the age historical, and thus inspire the comedy writers of future generations. This is more than evidenced in the wicked satires of Guyot de Provins (*Bible Guiot*), who cruelly assails the doctors; it was he who wrote the poem that said:

"Young doctors just come from Salern(o)

Sell blown-up bladders for lantern."

As we see, from perusing these numerous lampoons, physicians were not held in high esteem, notwithstanding the sacerdotal character in which the profession was invested. Meantime, in the *Roman du Noveau Renard*, we find a passage[4] that permits the supposition that physicians already possessed a certain amount of medical erudition; that they were acquainted with the works of Galen, and had full knowledge of all writers of the Arabian school, as well as that of the school of Salerno.

"Je faisoie le physicien

Et allegoie Galien,

Et montrois oeuvre ancienne

Et de Rasis et d'Avicenne,

Et a tous les faisoie entendre

In'estoie drois physiciens

Et maistre des practiciens."

In revenge, the author of the "Romance of Renard" accords but little confidence to medical art, for he adds very maliciously:

"All belief in medicine is folly,

Trust it and you lose your life;

For it is a fact most melancholy—

Where one is cured two perish in the strife."

Why the poet of the *Roman du Renard* was so full of rancor against the doctors of his time is a problem too difficult to solve; yet, while he considered them no better than criminals and dangerous men to society, he did not fail to call a doctor before dying. Physicians, for some strange and unknown reason, have always been criticised by French literary men in modern as well as ancient times. Our French authors have never, as did the masters of Greek poesy, recognized us as brothers in Apollo. Permit me here to call their attention to one of the writers of Greek anthology, who said of physicians:

"The son of Phœbus himself, Æsculapius, has instilled into thy mind, O Praxagorus, the knowledge of that divine art which makes care to be forgotten. He has given into thy hands the balm that cures all evils. Thou, too, hast learned from the sweet Epion what pains accompany long fevers, and the remedies to be applied to divided flesh; if mortals possessed medicines such as thine, the ferry of Charon would not be overloaded in crossing the Styx."

Notwithstanding sarcasm, in spite of epigrams and calumny, medicine has always been a source of sublime consolation to the sick and afflicted, the sufferer—rich and poor. At all ages the priest has been inclined to indulge in the practice of physic, and it was at their instigation that those nuns known as Sisters of Charity practiced medicine to a certain extent in the Middle Ages. In the twelfth century we see the nuns of the Convent of Paraclet, in Champagne, following the advice of Abelard, essaying the surgical treatment of the sick. It is true the first abbess of this nunnery was Heloise, in whose history conservative surgery is not even mentioned. The nuns who dressed wounds were called *medeciennes* or *miresses*. Gaulthier de Conisi has left a history of their good works:

"And the world wondered when it did learn

That woman had found a new mission;

When the doctors of Montpellier and Salern(o)

Saw each nun to be a physician.

A fever they knew, a pulse they could feel,

And best of it all is, *they managed to heal*."

This tendency of women to care for the sick now became general. "In our ancient poets and romancers," says Roquefort, "we often notice how young girls[5] were employed to cure certain wounds, because they were more tender-hearted and gentle-handed; as, for example, Gerard de Nevers, having been wounded, was carried into a chapel, where "a beautiful maiden took him in hand to effect a cure, and he thought so much of her that in brief space of time he commenced to mend; and was so much better that he could eat and drink; and he had such confidence in the skill of the maiden that, before a month passed, he was most perfectly cured."

As early as the sixth century, we note in the recital, *Des Temps Merovingiens*, by Augustin Thierry, that Queen Radegond, wife of Clotaire I., transformed her royal mansion into a hospital for indigent women. "One of the Queen's pastimes was to go thither not simply to visit, but to perform all the most repulsive duties of nurse."

In Feudal times it was the custom to educate the girls belonging to the nobility in practical medicine; also in surgery, especially that variety of surgery applied to wounds. This was immensely useful, inasmuch as their fathers, brothers, husbands or lovers were gallant "Knights," who ofttimes returned from combat or tourney mutilated or crippled. It was the delicate hand of titled ladies that rendered similar service to strange foreign knights who might be brought wounded to the castle gates. This is why the knights of old rendered such devout homage to the gentler sex—knowing their kindness and love in time of distress, when bleeding wounds were to be staunched and fever allayed. In a Troubadour song, *Ancassin et Nicolette*, we find this passage:

"Nicolette, in great alarm,

Asked about his pain;

Found out of joint his arm,

Put it in again;

Dressed with herbs the aching bone—

Plants to her had virtues known."

Although the church was hostile to the philosophy of Aristotle, whose works were publicly burned in 1209 A.D. by order of the Council, Pierre de Vernon published, in the same thirteenth century, a short poem by the title *Les Enseignements d'Aristote*, the object of which was to vulgarize the scientific portion of the great Greek author's Encyclopedia. This treatise commenced as follows:

"Primes saciez ke icest tretiez

- 6 -

Est le secre de secrez numez,

Ke Aristotle le Philosophe y doine,

La fiz Nichomache de Macedoine

A sun deciple Alisandre en bone fei,

Le grant, le fiz, a Philippe le Rei,

Le fist en sa graunt vielesce."

Which, translated from old French, reads: "From whence learn that this treatise is the secret of secrets, that Aristotle the philosopher, son of Nichomachus, gave to his pupil, Alexander the Great, son of King Philip, and which was composed in his old age."

In recalling the fact that Aristotle was the son of Nichomachus, Pierre de Vernon probably desired to call the attention of his readers more to the knowledge of medicine that the author derived from his father, the celebrated physician, than to the brilliant pupil of Plato.

Among the interesting passages in this poem we distinguish some that advise abstinence to persons whose maladies are engendered by excesses at table:

"One man cannot live without wine,

While another without it should dine;

For the latter, 'tis clear,

All grape juice and beer

For his own stomach's sake should decline."

The author claims drinking at meals induces gastralgia from acidity of the stomach:

"The signs of bad stomach thus trace:

Poor digestion, a red bloated face,

With out-popping eyes,

Palpitation, and sighs.

With oppression, as though one did lace."

He mentions eructations and sour belching as indicating frigidity of the stomach, and advises the drinking of very hot water before meals. Aside from this, he gives good counsel relative to all the advantages of a sober and peaceful life:

"If passion within you wax hot,

Pray don't eat and drink like a sot.

Give wine no license;

From rich food abstinence;

And luxurious peace is your lot."

The author then advises that the mouth and gums be well taken care of, that the teeth be neatly cleaned after each meal, and the entire buccal cavity be rinsed out with an infusion of bitter-sweet plants or leaves.

"Puis apres si froterez

Vos dents et gencives assez,

Od les escorces tut en tur

D' arbre chaud, sec. amer de savur

Kar iceo les dents ennientit," etc.

Notwithstanding their want of scientific form, these precepts still strongly contrast with the superstitious practices employed by the monks in the treatment of disease. When holy relics failed the priesthood had resource to supernatural power; they believed in the faith cure; the touch of a Royal hand could heal disease. They took all their scrofulous and goitre patients to Phillip I. and to Saint Louis. These sovereigns had not always an excessive faith in the miraculous gifts they were desired to bestow, but reasons of State policy forced them to accept this monkish deceit, which was regularly practiced by the clergy every Pentecost Day.

The *mise en scene* was easily arranged: the King of France, after holy communion at Saint Francis Convent, left the building surrounded by men at arms and Benedictine friars; then he touched the spots on his people, saying to each of his afflicted subjects: "*Rex tangit te, Deus sanat te, in nomine Patris et filii et Spiritus sancti.*"[6]

Block pretends that the King of England also enjoyed the power of curing epilepsy, and remarks *apropos* to this fact that the invention is not new, since Pyrrhus, King of Epirus, possessed the power of curing individuals attacked by enlarged spleen by simply pressing his right foot on that viscera.

But this is no longer a superstition to-day, since the age of miracles is past and the divinity of kings a belief almost without a disciple. However, Gilbert and Daniel Turner, physicians of the thirteenth century, give it credence in their writings, but they are fully entitled to express their independent opinion.

The priests of the Middle Ages could not employ themselves as obstetricians, neither could they treat uterine diseases. The *ventrieres* were the only midwives of the period; these women were allowed to testify as experts in the courts of justice, but the burden of proof rested on the testimony of at least three *sage femmes* when a newly-married woman was accused of pregnancy by a husband, as witness the following:

"Should a man declare his wife just wedded be pregnant and she deny the charge, it is well to conduct the accused woman to the house of some prudent female friend, and then that three *ventrieres* be summoned who may regard the suspect. If they declare her to be in a family way, the provost shall call the midwives as witnesses as before stated; but if the *sage femmes* declare the accused is not pregnant, then shall the wife have cause against her husband; but better is it when the husband, seeing the wrong wrought, shall humble himself and beg pardon."

Midwives were sworn, according to statutes and ordinances, which contained formulæ reports to be presented to the judges, to visit girls who complained of having been raped; fourteen signs of such deflowerment were admitted in testimony. Laurent Joubert has transcribed three of such reports, of which we will reproduce only one that was addressed to the Governor of Paris on October 23d, 1672:

"We, Marie Miran, Christophlette Reine, and Jeannie Porte, licensed midwives of Paris, certify to whom it may concern, that on the 22d day of October in the present year, by order of the Provost of Paris, of date 15th of aforesaid month, we visited a house in Rue Pompierre and there examined a girl aged thirty years, named Olive Tisserand, who had made complaint against one Jaques Mudont Bourgeois, whom she insisted deflowered her by violence. We examined the plaintiff by sight and the finger, and found as follows:

"Her breasts relaxed from below the neck downwards; *mammæ marcidæ et flaccidæ*; her vulva chafed; *os pubis collisum*; the hair on the os pubis curled; *pubes in orbem finuata*; the perineum wrinkled; *perinæum corrugatum*; the nature of the woman lost; *vulva dissoluta et mercessans*; the lips of private pendant; *labia pendenta*; the lesser lips slightly peeled; *labiorum oræ pilis defectæ*; the nymphæ depressed; *nymphæ depressæ*; the caroncles softened; *carunculæ dissolutæ*; the membrane connecting the caroncles retracted; *membrana connecteus inversa*; the clitoris was excoriated; *clitoris excoriata*; the uterine neck turned; *collum uteri*; the vagina distended; *finus pudoris*; in fact, the lady's hymen is missing; *hymen deductum*; finally, the internal orifice of the womb is open; *os internum matricis*. Having viewed this sad state of affairs, sign by sign, we have found traces *omnibus figillatum perspectis et perforutatis*, etc., and the above-named midwives certify to the before-mentioned Provost that the aforesaid statement under oath is true."

Physicians were not obliged by the magistrates to determine the nature of rapes on women; all gynecological questions were remanded to midwives. In truth, among all the physicians of antiquity only Hippocrates discussed uterine complaints and Ætius studied obstetrics. It was only in the sixteenth century that midwifery took its place among the medical sciences, thanks to Rhodion, Ambroise Parè, Reif, Rousset, and Guillemeau. Shortly before this time, that is to say, in the fifteenth century, Jacques de Foril published his "Commentaires" on generation, his ideas being derived from Avicenna; his notions, however, were absurd, being wholly based on astrological considerations. He pretended that an infant is not viable in the eighth month, because in the first month the pregnant woman is protected by Jupiter, from whom comes life; and in the seventh month by the moon, which favorizes life by its humidity and light; while in the eighth month or reign of Saturn, who eats children, the influence is hostile. But on the ninth month the benevolent influence of Jupiter is again experienced, and for this reason the infant is more apt to be alive at this period of gestation.

To the scholastic philosophy of the Middle Ages we must attribute the prejudice that, the human body being in direct connection with the universe, especially the planets, it was impossible for physical change to occur without the influence of the constellations. Thus astrology came to be considered as an essential part of medicine. This belief in the influence of the stars came from the Orient, and was carried through Europe after the crusades.

As to the treatise on "Diseases of Women," attributed to Trotula, a midwife of the school of Salerno, it is only a formulary of receipts for the use of women—baths in the sea-sands under a hot sun to thin ladies suffering from overfat; signs by which a good wet-nurse may be recognized: a method of kneading the head, the nose, and the limbs of new-born children before placing them in swaddling clothes; the use of virgin wine mixed with honey as a remedy for removing the wrinkles of old age.

"The *Commentaires* of Bernard de Provincial informs us," says Daremberg, "that certain practices, not only superstitious but disgusting, were common among the doctrines of Salerno; one, for instance, was to eat themselves, and also oblige their husbands to eat, the excrement of an ass fried in a stove in order to prevent sterility; likewise, to eat the stuffed heart of a diseased sow in order to forget dead friends," etc.

We can form some judgment, from such observations, as to the *therapeutic* wisdom of these doctrines of the school of Salerno. It is true, however, that at this epoch but little medicine save that of an unique and fantastic order was prescribed. Gilbert, the Englishman, advised, with the greatest British *sang froid*, tying a pig to the bed of a patient attacked by lethargy; he ordered lion's flesh in case of apoplexy, also scorpion's oil and angle-worm eggs; to dissolve stone in the bladder, he prescribed the blood of a young billy-goat nourished on diuretic herbs.

Peter of Spain, who was archbishop, and afterwards Pope, under the name of John XXI., was a man whom historians claim was more celebrated as a physician than as Pope; it was this Peter who adapted the curious medical formulary known by the title of *Circa Instans*, and, had improved on the invention. Those who wore on their bodies the words "Balthazar," "Gaspar" and "Melchior" need never fear attacks of epilepsy; in order to produce a flux in the belly, it was only necessary to put a patient's excrement in a human bone and throw it into a stream of water.

Hugo de Lucgnes, in fractures of the bone, employed a powder composed of ginger and cannella, which he used in connection with the "Lord's Prayer," in the meantime also invoking the aid of the Trinity. He treated hernia by cauterization, and leprosy by inunctions of mercurial ointment.

If therapeutics made only slight progress in the thirteenth century, we cannot say as much for other branches of the medical and natural sciences.

Arnauld de Villeneuve, physician, chemist and astrologer, particularly distinguished himself by discovering sulphuric, nitric and hydrochloric acids, and also made the first essence of turpentine.

Lanfranc attracted large numbers of students to the College of Saint Come, and exhibited his skill as an anatomist and surgeon. In one of his publications he gives a very remarkable description of chancres and other venereal symptoms.

At the Faculty of Montpellier, which was founded in 1220 A.D., we see as the Dean Roger of Parma, and as professor Bernard de Gordon, who left a very accurate account of leprosy and a number of observations on chancres following impure connection; these observations are valuable, inasmuch as they are corroborated by Lanfranc and his contemporary, Guillaume de Saliceto, of Italy, *two centuries before the discovery of America.*

Albert the Great (Albertus Magnus) and Roger Bacon also belonged to the thirteenth century.

Albert de Ballstatt, issue of a noble family of Swabia, monk of the order of St. Dominicus, after studying in the principal schools of Italy and Germany, arrived at Paris in 1222 A.D., and soon had numerous auditors, among whom may be mentioned Saint Augustin, Roger Bacon, Villeneuve, and other distinguished men. His lectures attracted such crowds of students from the University that he was obliged to speak from a public place in the Latin Quarter, which, in commemoration of his success, was called *Place Maitre Albert*, afterwards corrupted to Place Maubert.

His writings were encyclopedic, their principal merit being commentaries on the works of Aristotle, of whom but little was known at that period; he studied also the Latin translations of the Arabian school, and reviewed Avicenna and Averrhoes, adding to such works some original observations.

Albert the Great, or Albertus Magnus, the name posterity has bestowed on this genius, was also much occupied with alchemy, and passed for a magician. He was considered a sorcerer by many, as he was said to evoke the spirits of the departed, and produced wonderful phenomena.

Albert's works on natural history, his botany and mineralogy are, in reality, taken from the works of Aristotle, as well as his *parva naturalis*, which is only a reproduction of the *Organon* of the Greek philosopher; nevertheless, Albert deserves credit for his good work in relighting the torch of science in the Occident.

His disciple, Roger Bacon, was also a monk; he studied in Paris and afterwards removed to Oxford, England, where he actively devoted himself to natural science, especially physics. He left behind him remarkable observations on the refraction of light; explanation of the formation of rainbows, inventing the magnifying glass and telescope. His investigations in alchemy led him to discover a combustible body similar to phosphorus, while his work on "Old Age" (*De retardtandus senectutis occidentibus*) entitled him to a high position among the physicians of the thirteenth century. Although one of the founders of experimental science, one of the initiators—if the expression may be used—of scientific positivism, he also devoted much time to astrology. Denounced as a magician and sorcerer by his own *confreres* in religion, he was condemned to perpetual imprisonment, and was only released a few years before his death, leaving many writings on almost every branch of science.

It was more than a century after these two great men died that medical science commenced its upward flight.

Anatomy, proscribed by the Catholic Church, had an instant's toleration in the middle of the thirteenth century, thanks to the protection of Frederick II., King of the Two Sicilies. But an edict of Pope Boniface VIII., published in 1300, forbid dissections once more, not only in Italy, but in all countries under Papal rule. Nevertheless, in 1316, Mondinus, called the restorer of anatomy, being professor at the University of Bologna, had the courage to dissect the cadavers of two patients in public; he then published an account of the same, which Springer declares had "the advantage of having been made after nature, and which is preferable to all works on anatomy published since Galen's time."

Some years later the prejudice against human dissection disappeared in France, and anatomy was allowed to be taught by the Faculties of Paris and Montpellier. Henri de Hermondaville, Pierre de Cerlata, and Nicholas Bertrucci were particularly distinguished anatomists during the fourteenth century, and traced the scientific path followed by Vesalius, Fallopius, Eustachius, Fabrica de Aguapendente, Sylvius, Plater, Varola de Torre, Charles Etienne, Ingrassias, and Arantius in the sixteenth century.

From this time dates the escape of medicine from ecclesiastical authority.

In 1452, Cardinal d'Estouteville, charged by the Pope with the reorganization of the University of Paris, obtained a revocation of the order obliging celibacy, claiming it to be "impious and senseless" in the case of doctors.

It was at this moment that the Faculty of Physicians renounced the hospitality of the University and installed themselves in a house on the *Rue de la Bucherie*, the same being graciously tendered them by Jacques Desparts, physician to the King. This faculty now opened a register of its acts, which later became the *Commentaries of the Society*, and, already confident of a brilliant future and its own strength, the college engraved on its escutcheon these words: "*Urbi et Orbi Salus*," and declared itself the guardian of antique morality; *veteris disciplinæ retinentissima*. Soon the dean of the faculty obtained from royalty the right to coin medals, the same being bestowed on physicians who rendered valuable public services; these bore the imprint of the college coat of arms, and Guy Patin went so far as to issue his own coined effigy in 1632 A.D.

The royal authority still further aided the medical profession and the faculty in gathering students: for instance, an order was issued granting physicians titles of nobility and coats of arms in cases of great merit; they were also exempted from taxes and other contributions to the crown, for, says Louis XIV., who speaks, "We cannot withhold such marks of honor to men of learning and others who by their devotion to a noble profession and personal merit are entitled to a rank of high distinction." Besides, some of the greatest names in France were inscribed on the registers of the faculty; let us cite, for instance, Prader, Mersenne, Saint Yon, Montigny, Mauvillain, Sartes, Revelois, Montrose, Farcy, Jurency, and others. Can it be astonishing that the Faculty of Medicine, considering such high favors, was so deeply attached to the royalty that gave liberty and reputation to the great thinkers of the age?

The dean, who before the thirteenth century only had the title *Magister Scolarum*, administered the affairs of the faculty without control, and was recognized as the chief hierarch of the corporation; but he was elected by all the professors, and often chosen outside the professors of the Faculty. This high office was thus duly dignified, and it was only justice.

Above the dean, however, was the first Physician to the King, who was a high officer of the crown, having the same rights and privileges as the nobility, securing on his appointment the title of Count with hereditary transmission of same to his family; he was also a Councillor of State and wore the costume and decorations of this order. When he came to the faculty meetings he was received by the dean and bachelors, for he was also grand master of hygiene and legal medicine in the realm; he named all the salaried medical appointments, notably those of experts in medical jurisprudence.

Under Charles VIII., Adam Fumee and Jean Michel, sitting in Parliament as Councillors; Jacques Coictier, physician to Louis XI., was the President of the Tax Commission; while Fernel, no less celebrated as a mathematician than as a physician, was the intimate friend of Henri II. at the same time that Ambroise Pare was surgeon to the latter King and his two successors; F. Miron, too, afterwards became Embassador to Henri III.

Later we see Vautier, physician to *Marie de Medecis*, one of the malcontents sent to the Bastile for political reasons. Valot, Daquin and Fagon, all physicians to Louis XIV., were politicians, but were also great dispensers of Royal favor. Medical politicians figured largely in the time of Louis XIV. Among the independents, we may cite Guy Patin, the intimate friend and adviser of Lamoignan and Gabriel Naude, who was one of the most erudite men of the age. Under such conditions, no wonder that medicine entered into a new phase of progress. The time of study was now fixed at six years; after this there were examinations, from which, unfortunately, however, clinical medicine was excluded; examinations corresponded with the grades of Bachelor and doctor; finally—triumphant act of culmination—came the thesis with the obligation of the solemn Hippocratic oath.

The degree of Bachelor had existed since the foundation of the University of Paris. The Bacchalauri, or Bachalarrii,[7] were always students for the doctoral title. After numerous other tests, they signed the following obligation:

1. I swear to faithfully observe all secrets with honor, to follow the code and statutes laid down by the Faculty, and to do all in my power to assist them.

2. I swear to always obey and respect the Dean of the Faculty.

3. I swear to aid the Faculty in resisting any undertaking against their honor or ordinances, especially against those so-called doctors who practice illicitly; and also submit to any punishment inflicted for a proscribed action.

4. I swear to assist in full robes, at all meetings, when ordered by the Faculty.

5. I swear to assist at the exercises of the Academy of Medicine and the school for the space of two years, and sustain any question assigned me, in medicine or hygiene, by a thesis. Finally, I swear to be a good citizen, loving peace and order, and observe a decent manner in discussion on all questions laid down by the Faculty.

This oath was read in Latin by the Dean, and, as enumerated, each candidate for a degree solemnly answered "I swear" after each article.

Ranged with physicians at this period, although on a lower plane, came the surgeons and barbers; these had been created under the title of *mires* and *meges*, by medical monks, who could not, under the canons, resort to surgical operations, as it is written *Ecclesia abhorrhet a sanguine*.

Let us continue their history. When the College of Physicians was added to the University of Paris, in the twelfth century, it was specified by the other Faculties of the institution that surgeons formed no portion of the medical Faculty, and were not entitled to any consideration. These surgeons kept shops and wandered through the streets with instrument cases on their backs, seeking clients, and were assisted in their work by the barbers, who were even more illiterate than the surgeons; but, thanks to the exertions of Jean Pitard, surgeon to Saint Louis, these surgeons succeeded in forming a corporation in 1271. Their meetings were held in the dead-house of the Cordeliers' church, and they were allowed the same privileges as the *magistri in physica*. They were the surgeons wearing a long robe.

It was only at the end of the century that Lanfranc obtained from Phillip the Beautiful an order to reorganize and bestow degrees for the exercise of surgical art. The studies were extremely practical; they required several years' attendance at the Hotel Dieu or in the service of some city surgeon, likewise a certain amount of literary education. Like the doctors, these surgeons were permitted to wear a robe and hat. They were a great success.

Unfortunately, the barbers of the fourteenth century obtained, in their turn, an edict from Charles V., who recognized their corporation and authorized the knights of the razor to practice bleeding, and also all manner of minor surgery.

The Faculty of Medicine, jealous of the Surgeons' College, encouraged the barbers with all their influence. They founded for the face scrapers a special course in anatomy on condition that the barber would always acknowledge the physician as superior to the surgeon. The barbers made this promise, but the time arrived when they thought themselves stronger than the Faculty of Medicine; this was in 1593; but this same year, an order passed by Parliament, at the instigation of the doctors, deprived the barbers of all the power granted them by Charles V.

The barbers thus had their punishment for defying the Faculty of Medicine.

The College of Surgeons, relieved from the competition of the barber surgeons, now claimed the right to become part of the Medical Faculty, and an ordinance of Francois I. gave them this privilege. Letters patent were issued that read:

"It is ordained that the before-mentioned, professors, bachelors, licentiates or masters, be they married or single, shall enjoy all the privileges, franchises, liberties, immunities and exemptions accorded to the other medical graduates of the University."

Notwithstanding this Royal edict and confirmation of privileges accorded to surgeons by Henri II., Charles IX., and Henri III., the Faculty of Medicine positively refused to open their doors to their mortal enemies, the much despised barber-surgeons, as they were termed.

Even Louis XIV. gave up the idea of making the doctors associate socially with the surgeons; the latter, then, continued to keep shops, with a sign of three sacrament boxes supported by a golden lily, and were only allowed the cadavers of malefactors for purposes of dissection; these bodies were stolen from the Faculty of Medicine. In the meantime, the regular barber-surgeons renewed their ancient allegiance to the doctors, who had vainly attempted to substitute students in their places.

To put an end to the struggle, the College of Surgeons took the desperate but injurious resolve to admit all barbers to their institution and recognize their rights to a surgical degree. A year later, 1660, the Faculty of Medicine demanded that, inasmuch as the College of Surgeons admitted ignorant barbers to their school, the right of surgeons to wear a medical robe and hat and bestow degrees be denied. The Faculty of medicine gained their suit.

As an indispensable adjunct to the doctor at this period, let us now mention the apothecary and the bath-keeper.

The patron of the apothecaries was Saint Nicholas; they belonged to the corporation of grocers, where they were represented by three members. Their central bureau was at the Cloister Saint Opportune.

The inspection of drug stores and apothecary shops in Paris occurred once a year, and was made by three members elected from the central bureau and two doctors in medicine. A druggist in Paris served four years as an apprentice and six years as an under-dispenser; then the applicant was obliged to pass two examinations, and, finally, five extra examinations, the latter in the presence of the master apothecaries and two doctors. Notwithstanding their oath[8] to not prescribe medicine for the sick and not to sell drugs without a doctor's written order, druggists then, as now, had frequent conflicts with physicians, as the latter are ever jealous of non professional interference and always asserting supremacy.

However, it is well to say that druggists never violated the rule relative to strict inspection of all drugs before using such articles. All medicines were passed at the central bureau before any apothecary would purchase for dispensing purposes.

As to bath-keepers, they belonged in antique times, as now, more to the order of empirics; their history dates far back to the period when the Romans introduced their bathing system into Gaul—a system which was perpetuated up to as late as the sixteenth century.

The baths constructed by the ancients and destroyed by the barbarians, reappeared again in the Middle Ages, under the names of vapor baths and furnace baths. These baths were shops, usually kept by barbers, where one could be sheared, sweated or leeched by a tonsorial artist. All the world then took baths—even the monks washed themselves sometimes; in fact, almost every monastery had its bath-rooms, where the poor could wash and be bled without pay.

In those days gentlemen bathed before receiving the order of chivalry. When one gave a ball it was customary and gallant to offer all the guests, especially the ladies, a free bath. When Louis XI. went out to sup with his loyal subjects, the honest tradespeople of Paris, he always found a hot bath at his disposal. Finally, it was considered a severe penance to forbid a person from bathing, as was done in the case of Henry IV., who was excommunicated.

Paris had many bath-houses. From early dawn until sunset the streets were filled, with cryers for bath-houses, who invited all passers-by to enter. In the time of Charles VI., bath-keepers introduced vapor baths. Some of these latter were entirely given up to women; others were reserved for the King and gentlemen of the court. The price of vapor baths was fixed by Police ordinance at twenty centimes for a vapor bath and forty centimes for those who washed afterwards. This price was subject to revision only at the pleasure of the municipal authorities.

During times of epidemics vapor baths were discontinued. It was for sanitary reasons, probably, that an order of the Mayor of Paris, named Delamere, forbade all persons taking vapor baths until after Christmas eve, "on penalty of a heavy fine." This same proclamation was repeated by act of Parliament on December 13th, 1553, "the penalty corporeal punishment for offending bath-keepers."

Parisian vapor baths had such wide-spread reputations and success that an Italian doctor of the sixteenth century by the name of Brixanius, who arrived in Paris, wrote the following verses:

"Balnea si calidis queras sudantia thermis,

In claris intrabis aqua, ubi corpus inungit,

Callidus, et multo medicamine spargit aliptes',

Mox ubi membra satis geminis mundata lacertis

Laverit et sparsos crines siccaverit, albo

Marcida subridens componit corpora lecto."

Already, in the time of Saint Louis, the number of bath-keepers was so great that they had a trades union; they were almost all barbers, too; they washed the body, cut hair, trimmed corns and nails, shaved and leeched.

Bath houses more than multiplied from the twelfth century, imitations of Oriental customs, due to the crusaders. Baths were run not only by men, but by old harridans and fast girls. No respectable woman ever entered a public bath-house; Christine de Pisan bears witness to that fact in the following lines: "As to public baths and vapor baths, they should be avoided by honest women except for good cause; they are expensive and no good comes out of them, for many obvious reasons; no woman, if she be wise, would trust her honor therein, if she desire to keep it."

The establishments known as vapor baths, as early as the time of Saint Louis, had already degenerated into houses of prostitution. The police, in defense of public morality, were finally obliged to forbid fast women and diseased men from frequenting such places.

In Italy, vapor baths were recognized officially and tolerated as places of public debauchery; this was also the case in Avignon. The Synodal statutes of the Church of Avignon, in the year 1441, bear an ordinance drawn by the civil magistrates and applicable to married men and also to priests and clergy, forbidding access to the vapor baths on the Troucat Bridge, which were set apart as a place of tolerated debauchery by the municipal authorities. This ordinance contained a provision that was very uncommon in the Middle Ages, *i.e.*, a fine of ten marks for a violation of the law during day time and twenty marks fine for a violation occurring under cover of night.

In 1448 the city council of Avignon again tried its hand at regulating the vapor baths at the bridge; but the golden days of debauched women had long before passed away, and the previous century had witnessed the acme of the courtesans' fortunes. The sojourn of the Popes at Avignon had gathered together from all over the Globe a motley collection of pilgrims and begotten a frightful condition of libertinage; we have the authority of Petrarch in saying that it even surpassed that of the Eternal City, and Bishop Guillaume Durand presented the Council of Vienna with a graphic picture of this social evil.

According to the proclamation of Etienne Boileau, Mayor of Paris in the reign of Louis IX., barber bath keepers were forbidden to employ women of bad reputation in their shops in order to carry on under cover, as in the massage shops of the present day, an infamous commerce, on penalty of losing their outfit—seats, basins, razors, etc.,—which were to be sold at public auction for the profit of the public treasury and the Crown. But we know full well that the Royal Ordinance of 1254, which had for its object the reformation of public debauchery, was only applied for the space of two years, and that the new law of 1256 re-established and legalized public prostitution which offered less objectionable features than clandestine prostitution.

The use of public baths and hydrotherapy lasted until the sixteenth century. At this epoch, and without any known reason, the public suddenly discontinued all balneary practices, and this was noticeable among the aristocratic class as among the common people. A contrary evil was developed. "Honest women," says Vernille, "took a pride in claiming that they never permitted themselves certain ablutions." Nevertheless, Marie de Romien, (*Instruction pour les Jeunes Dames*) in her classical work for the instruction of young women, remarks: "They should keep clean, if it be only for the satisfaction of their husbands; it is not necessary to do as some women of my acquaintance, who have no care to wash until they be foul under their linen. But to be a beautiful *damoyselle* one may wash reasonably often in water which has been previously boiled and scented with fragrants, for nothing is more certain than that beauty flourishes best in that young woman who not only looks but smells clean."

In an opuscle published in 1530, by one called De Drusæ, we observe that "notwithstanding the natural laws of propriety, women use scents more than clean water; and they thus only increase the bad smells they endeavor to disguise. Some use greasy perfumed ointments, others sponges saturated in fragrants"

"Entre leur cuisses et dessoubz les aisselles,

Pour ne sentir l'espaulle de mouton."

This horror of water did not last long, however, and at the commencement of the seventeenth century the false modesty of women ended with the creation of river baths, such as exist to-day along the banks of the Seine.

Was this restoration of cleanly habits due to medical advice? This question cannot be answered, but it may not be out of place to cite that remarkable passage from the "Essays of Montaigne" on the hygiene of bathing, which he recommends in certain maladies:

"It is good to bathe in warm water, it softens and relaxes in ports where it stagnates over sands and stones. Such application of external heat, however, makes the kidneys leathery and hard and petrifies the matter within. To those who bathe: it is best to eat little at night to the end that the waters drank the next morning operate more easily, meeting with an empty stomach. On the other hand, it is best to eat a little dinner, in order not to trouble the action of the water, which is not in perfect accord; nor should the stomach be filled too suddenly after its other labor; leave the work of digestion to the night, which is better than the day, when the body and mind are in perpetual movement and activity.

"I have noted, on the occasion of my voyages, all the famous baths of Christendom, and for some years past have made use of waters, for as a general rule I consider bathing healthy and deem it no risk to one's physical condition. The custom of ablution, so generally observed at times past in all nations, is now only practiced in a few as a daily habit. I cannot imagine why civilized people ever allow their bodies to become encrusted with dirt and their pores filled with filth."[9]

If Montaigne made great use of mineral waters, he had in revenge a formidable dread of physicians and their medicines, a sentiment he inherited from his father, "who died," says he, "at the age of seventy-four years," and his "grandfather and great-grandfather died at eighty years without tasting a drop of physic."

Montaigne has justly criticized medicine in several essays on the healing art. He knew well the *intividia medicorum*, and it was for this reason that he remarked that a physician should always treat a case without a consultant. "There never was a doctor," says Montaigne, "who, on accepting the services of a consultant, did not discontinue or readjust something." Is not the same criticism deserved at the present day? How absurd are our medical consultations. The examples Montaigne gives of disagreements of doctors in consultation as to doctrines are equally applicable to modern times. The differences of Herophilus, Erasistratus, and the Æsclepiadæ as to the original causation of disease were no greater than those of the schools of Broussais and Pasteur, which have both acquired a universal celebrity in less than half a century.

Montaigne insisted that medicine owed its existence only to mankind's fear of death and pain, an impatience at poor health and a furious and indiscreet thirst for a speedy cure, but the author of the "Essays" adds in concluding: "I honor physicians, not following the feeling of necessity, but for the love of themselves, having seen many honest doctors who were honorable and well worthy of being loved."

The reputation for disagreement among doctors so much insisted on by Montaigne has served as a well-worn text for many other critics.

In *Les Serres* of Guillaume Bouchet, a contemporary of the author, we find the same shaft of sarcasm directed at physicians. Where will you find men in any other profession save that of medicine who envy and hate each other so heartily? What other profession on earth is given over to such bitter disagreements? How can common people be expected to honor and respect experts and savants so-called when the professors call each other ignoramusses and asses? Call these doctors into a case and one after the other they will disagree as to the diagnosis as well as to the method of cure. As Pellisson wrote:

"When an enemy you wish to kill

Don't call assasins full of vice,

But call two doctors of great skill

To give contrary advice."

Or in the verses of the original:

"D'un ennemi voulez vous defaire?

Ne cherchez pas d'assasins

Donnez lui deux medecins,

Et qui'ils soient d'avis contrarie."

This professional jealousy is always more apparent than real. Aside from the rivalry for public patronage physicians are a very social class of men, as witness their many festive meetings. We banquet in honor of St. Luke the physician, and St. Come, after each thesis, at anniversaries, at the election of the Dean, and on many other occasions. It is these co-fraternal meetings at which are reinagurated the old feelings of good-fellowship; our little quarrels only serve to discipline the medical body and to increase the grandeur of the Faculty. It is the constant rubbing of surfaces that makes the true professional metal glitter.

When we hear new doctors, young graduates, swear the Hippocratic oath, we do not forget that the principal articles of the statute prescribe the cultivation of friendships, respect for the older members of the profession, benevolence to the young beginners, and the preservation of professional decency and kindness. It may be insisted that banquets are not to be considered as medical assemblages, for there they laugh long and loud, and drink many a bumper of rich Burgundy; making joyous discourse; holding to the famous compliment of Moliere:

Salus, honor et argentum

Atque bonum appetitum.

We know to-day many of the truthful precepts of the School of Salerno and their bearing on the medical records of the middle ages. Then as now the doctor had the ever increasing ingratitude of the patient (*ad proccarendam oegrorum ingratitudinem*).

"The disciple of Hippocrates meeteth often treatment rude,

The payment of his trouble is base ingratitude.

When the patient is in grievous pain the time is opportune

For a keen, sharp-witted doctor to make a good fortune.

Let him profit by the sufferer's aches and gather in the money,

For the ant gets winter provender and the summer bee its honey."

Our ancient friends had no pity for charlatans, however. They rightfully abused all medical impostors, as we read in the precepts of Salerno's school:

"Il n'est par d'ignorant, de chartatan stupide,

D'histron imposteur, ou de Juif fourbe avide,

De sorciere crasseuse ou de barbier bavard,

De faussiare inpudent, ou de moine cafard,

De marchand de savon, ou de avengle oculiste,

De baigneur imbecile, ou d'absurde alchimiste,

Pas d'heretigue impur qui ne se targue, enfin,

Du beau titre, du nom sacre de medecin."

The investigation of medical science was far from being an honor to the middle ages. The best of the profession was hidden in the doctoral sanctuary, enveloped in those mysteries which are never penetrated by the profane and only known to the initiated.

The recommendations as to the secrets of our art are addressed to all young doctors in that famous epilogue commencing:

"Gardez surtout, gardez qui'un profane vulgaire

De votre art respecte ne perce le mystere;

Son eclat devoile perdrait sa dignite

D'un mystere connu decroit la majeste,"

Let us invoke God, the Supreme physician, let us demand the professional banishment of every doctor who reveals a professional secret.

"Exsul sit medicus physicius secreta revelans."—Amen!

THE GREAT EPIDEMICS OF THE MIDDLE AGES.

THE PLAGUE

Several great epidemics of the Plague had already devastated the world; the plague of Athens in the fifth century, B. C.; the plague of the second century, in the reign of Marcus Aurelius; the plague of the third century, in the reign of Gallus; then came that most terrible epidemic of the sixth century, known by the name of the inguinal pestilence, which, after ravaging Constantinople spread into Liguria, then into France and Spain. It was in 542, according to Procopius, that an epidemic struck the world and consumed almost all the human species.[10]

"It attacked the entire earth," says our author, "striking every race of people, sparing neither age nor sex; differences in habitation, diet, temperament or occupation of any nature did not stop its ravages; it prevailed in summer and in winter, in fact, at every season of the year.

"It commenced at the town of Pelusa in Egypt, from whence it spread by two routes, one through Alexandria and the rest of Egypt, the other through Palestine. After this it covered the whole world, progressing always by regular intervals of time and force. In the springtime of 543 it broke out in Constantinople and announced itself in the following manner:

"Many victims believed they saw the spirits of the departed rehabilitated in human form. It appeared as though these spirits appeared before the subject about to be attacked and struck him on certain portions of the body. These apparitions heralded the onset of the malady. It is but fair to say that the commencement of the disease was not the same in all cases. Some victims did not see the apparitions, but only dreamed of them, but all believed they heard a ghostly voice announcing their inscription on the list of those who were going to die. Some claim that the greater number of victims were not haunted either sleeping or waking by these ghosts and the mysterious voice that made sinister predictions.

"The fever at the onset of the attack came on suddenly,—some while sleeping, some while waking, some while at work. Their bodies exhibited no change of color, and the temperature was not very high. Some indications of fever were perceptible, but no signs of acute inflammation. In the morning and at night the fever was slight, and indicated nothing severe either to the patient or to the physician who counted the pulse. Most of those who presented such symptoms showed no indications of approaching dissolution; but the first day among some, the second day in others, and after several days in many cases, a bubo was observed on the lower portion of the abdomen, in the groin, or in the folds of the axilla, and sometimes back of the ears or on the thighs.

"The principal symptoms of the disease on its invasion were as I have pointed out; for the remainder, nothing can be precisely indicated of the variations of the type of the disease following temperament; these other symptoms were only such as were imprinted by the Supreme Being at his divine will.

"Some patients were plunged into a condition of profound drowsiness; others were victims to furious delirium. Those who were drowsy remained in a passive state, seeming to have lost all memory of the things of ordinary life. If they had any one to nurse them they took food when offered from time to time, and if they had no care soon died of inanition. The delirious patients, deprived of sleep, were eternally pursued by their hallucinations; they imagined themselves haunted by men ready to slay them, and they sought flight from such fancied foes, uttering dreadful screams. Persons who were attacked while nursing the sick were in the most pitiable condition— not that they were more liable to contract the disease by contact, however, for nurses and doctors did not get the disease from actual contact with the sufferers, for some who washed and laid out the dead never contracted the malady, but enjoyed perfect health throughout the epidemic; some, however, died suddenly without apparent cause. Many of the nurses were overworked keeping patients from rolling out of bed and preventing the delirious from jumping from high windows. Some patients endeavored to throw themselves in running water, not to quench their thirst, but because they had lost all reason. It was necessary to struggle with many of the sick in order to make them swallow any nourishment, which they would not accept without more or less resistance. The buboes enfeebled certain patients who were neither drowsy nor delirious, but who finally succumbed to their atrocious sufferings.

"As nothing was known of this strange disease, certain physicians thought its origin was due to some source of evil hidden in the buboes, and they accordingly opened these glandular bodies. The dissection of the bubo showed sub-adjacent carbuncles, whose rapid malignity brought on sudden death or an illness of but few days' duration. In some instances the entire body was covered by black spots the size of a bean. Such unfortunates rarely lived a day, and generally expired in an hour. Many cases died suddenly, vomiting blood. One thing I can solemnly affirm, that is, that the wisest physicians gave up all hope in the case of many patients who afterwards recovered; on the contrary, many persons perished at the very time their health was almost re-established. For all these causes, the malady passed the confines of human reasoning, and the outcome always deceived the most natural predictions.

"As to treatment, the effects were variable, following the condition of the victim. I may state that, as a fact, no efficacious remedies were discovered that could either prevent the onset of the disease or shorten its duration. The victims could not tell why they were attacked, nor how they were cured.

"Pregnant women attacked inevitably aborted at death, some succumbing while miscarrying; some going on to the end of gestation, dying in labor along with their infants. Only three cases are known where women recovered of plague after aborting; while only one instance is on record where a newly-born child survived its mother in this epidemic. Those in whom the buboes increased most rapidly in size, maturated and suppurated, most often recovered, for the reason, no doubt, that the malignant properties of the bubonic carbuncle were weakened or destroyed.

"Experience proved that such symptoms were an almost sure presage of a return to health. Those, on the contrary, in whom the tumor did not change its aspect from the time of its eruption, were attacked with all the symptoms I have before described. In some cases the skin dried and seemed thus to prevent the tumor, although it might be well developed, from suppurating. Some were cured at the price of a loss of power in the tongue, which reduced the victims to stammer and articulate words in a confused and unintelligible manner for the rest of their days.

"The epidemic at Constantinople lasted four months, three months of which time it raged with great violence. As the epidemic progressed the mortality-rate increased from day to day, until it reached the point of 5,000 deaths per day, and on several occasions ran up to as high as 10,000 deaths in the twenty four hours."

Let us pass over this very important description that Procopius gives of the moral effect of this epidemic on the people, of the scenes of wild and heart-rending terror, of curious examples of egotism and sublime devotion, of instances of blind superstition developed in a great city under the influence of fear and the dread of a very problematical contagion.

Evagre, the scholastic, another Greek historian of the sixth century, recounts in his works the story of the plague at Constantinople. He states that he frequently observed that persons recovering from a first and second attack subsequently died on a third attack; also that persons flying from an infected locality were often taken sick after many days of an incubating period, falling ill in their places of refuge in the midst of populations free, up to that time, from the pestilence.

In following the progress of this epidemic from the Orient to the Occident, it was noticed that it always commenced at the sea-ports and then traveled inland. The disease was carried much more easily by ships than it could be at the present time, inasmuch as there were no quarantines and no pest-houses for isolating patients. It entered France by the Mediterranean Sea. It was in 549 that the plague struck Gaul. "During this time," says Gregory of Tours, "the malady known as the *inguinal disease* ravaged many sections and the province of Arles was cruelly depopulated."[11]

This illustrious historian wrote in another passage: "We learned this year that the town of Narbonne was devastated by the *groin disease*, of so deadly a type that when one was attacked he generally succumbed. Felix, the Bishop of Nantes, was stricken down and appeared to be desperately ill. The fever having ceased, the humor broke out on his limbs, which were covered with pustules. It was after the application of a plaster covered with cantharides that his limbs rotted off, and he ceased to live in the seventieth year of his age.

"Before the plague reached Auvergne it had involved most all the rest of the country. Here the epidemic attacked the people in 567, and so great was the mortality that it is utterly impossible to give even the approximate number of deaths. Populations perished *en masse*. On a single Sunday morning three hundred bodies were counted in St. Peter's chapel at Clermont awaiting funeral service. Death came suddenly; it struck the axilla or groin, forming a sore like a serpent that bit so cruelly that men rendered up their souls to God on the second or third day of the attack, many being so violent as to lose their senses. At this time Lyons, Bourges, Chalons, and Dijon were almost depopulated by the pestilence."

In 590 the towns of Avignon and Viviers were cruelly ravaged by the *inguinal disease.*

The plague reached Marseilles, however, in 587, being carried there by a merchant vessel from Spain which entered the port as a center of an infection. Several persons who bought goods from this trading vessel, all of whom lived in one house nevertheless, were carried off by the plague to the number of eight. The spark of the epidemic did not burn very rapidly at first, but after a certain time the baleful fire of the pest, after smouldering slowly, burst out in a blaze that almost consumed Marseilles.

Bishop Theodorus isolated himself in a wing of the cloister Saint Victor, with a small number of persons who remained with him during the plague, and in the midst of their general desolation continued to implore Almighty God for mercy, with fasting and prayer until the end of the epidemic. After two months of calm the population of the city commenced to drift back, but the plague reappeared anew and most of those who returned died. The plague has devastated Marseilles many times since the epoch just mentioned.

Anglada[12] who, like the writer, derives most of his citations from Gregory of Tours, thinks that the plague that devastated Strasbourg in 591 was only the same *inguinal disease* that ravaged Christendom. He cites, in support of his assertion, that passage from the historian poet Kleinlande translated by Dr. Boersch: "In 591 there was a great mortality throughout our country, so that men fell down dying in the streets, expiring suddenly in their houses, or even at business. When a person sneezed his soul was apt to fly the body; hence the expression on sneezing, 'God bless you!' And when a person yawned they made the sign of the cross before their mouths."

Such are the documents we possess on the great epidemic of inguinal plague of the fourth century, documents furnished by historians, to whom medical history is indebted, and not from medical authors, who left no marks at that period.

THE BLACK PLAGUE.

The Black Plague of the fourteenth century was more destructive even than the bubonic pest of the sixth century, and all other epidemics observed up to the present day. In the space of four years more than twenty five millions of human beings perished—one-half the population of the world. Like all other pestilences, it came from the Orient—from India, and perhaps from China. Europe was invaded from east to west, from south to north. After Constantinople, all the islands and shores of the Mediterranean were attacked, and successively became so many foci of disease from which the pestilence radiated inland. Constantinople lost two-thirds of its population. Cyprus and Cairo counted 15,000 deaths. Florence paid an awful tribute to the disease, so great being the mortality that the epidemic has often been called *Peste de Florence*; "100,000 persons perished," says Boccaccio. Venice lost 20,000 victims, Naples 60,000, Sicily 53,000, and Genoa 40,000, while in Rome the dead were innumerable.

In Spain, Germany, England, Poland, and Russia the malady was as fatal as in Italy. At London they buried 100,000 persons in the cemeteries. It was the same in France. Avignon lost 150,000 citizens in seven months, among whom was the beautiful Laura de Noves, immortalized by Petrarch, who expired from the plague in 1348, aged forty-one years. At Marseilles 56,000 people died in one month; at Montpellier three quarters of the population, including all the physicians, went down in the epidemic. Narbonne had 30,000 deaths and Strasbourg 16,000 in the first year of the outbreak. Paris was not spared; the *Chronique de Saint Denis* informs us that "in the year of Grace 1348, commenced the aforesaid mortality in the Realms of France, the same lasting about a year and a half, increasing more and more until Paris lost each day 800 inhabitants; so that the number who died there amounted to more than 500,000 people, while in the town of Saint Denis the number reached 16,000.[13]

Among the victims were Jeanne de Bourgogne, wife of Philip VI.; Jeanne II., Queen of Navarre, grandchild of Philip the Beautiful. In Spain, died Alphonse XI. of Castille. "Happily," says the *Chronicle*, "during the years following the plague the fecundity of women was prodigious—as though nature desired to repair the ravages wrought by death." The symptoms and history of this plague have been described by several ocular witnesses, among others Guy de Chauliac, the celebrated surgeon and professor at Montpellier, who has left the following recital in quaint old French:

"The disease was such that one never before saw a like mortality. It appeared in Avignon in the year of our Saviour 1348, in the sixth year of the Pontificate of Clement VI., in whose service I entered, thanks to his Grace.

"Not to displease you, I shall briefly narrate for your edification the advent of the disease.

"It commenced—the aforesaid mortality—in January and lasted for the space of seven months.

"The disease was of two kinds. The first type lasted two months, with a continued fever and spitting of blood. This variety killed in three days, however.

"The second type of the disease, prevailing during the epidemic time, also had a continued fever, with apostumes and carbuncles at the external parts, principally on the axilla and in the groin; all such attacked usually died in five days.

"The malady was so contagious, especially that form in which blood-spitting was noticed, that one not only caught it from sojourning with the sick, but also, it sometimes seemed, from looking at the disease, so that men died without their servants and were buried without priests.

"The father visited not his son, nor the son his father. Charity was dead and hope disappeared.

"I call the epidemic great, inasmuch as it conquered all the earth.

"For the pestilence commenced at the Orient, and cast its fangs against all the world, passing through Paris towards the West.

"It was so destructive that it left only a quarter of the population of mankind behind.

"It was a shame and disgrace to medicine, as many doctors dared not visit the sick through fear of becoming infected; and those who visited the sick made few cures and fewer fees, for the sick all died save a few. Not many having buboes escaped death.

"For preservation, there was no better remedy than to fly from the infection, to purge one's self with aloe pills, to diminish the blood by phlebotomy, to purify the air with fire, to comfort the heart with cordials and apples and other things of good odor; to console the humors with Armenian bole and resist dry rot by the use of acid things. For the cure of the plague we used bleedings and evacuations, electuaries, syrups and cordials, and the external apostumes or swellings were poulticed with boiled figs and onions mixed with oil and butter; the buboes were afterwards opened and treated by the usual cures for ulcers.

"Carbuncles were leeched, scarified and cauterized.

"I, to avoid infamy, dared not absent myself from the care of the sick, but lived in continual fear, preserving myself as long as possible by the before-mentioned remedies.

"Nevertheless, towards the end of the epidemic, I fell into a fever, which continued with an aposthume in the groin, and was ill for nigh on six weeks, being in such danger that all my companions believed I should die; nevertheless, the bubo being poulticed and treated as I have above indicated, I recovered, thanks be to the will of God."

According to the records of that time, many persons died the first day of their illness. These bad cases were announced by a violent fever, with cephalgia, vertigo, drowsiness, incoherency in ideas, and loss of memory; the tongue and palate were black and browned, exhaling an almost insupportable fetidity. Others were attacked by violent inflammation of the lungs, with hemorrhage; also gangrene, which manifested itself in black spots all over the body; if, to the contrary, the body was covered by abscesses, the patients seemed to have some chance for recovery.

Medicines were powerless, all remedies seeming to be useless. The disease attacked rich and poor indiscriminately; it overpowered the robust and debilitated; the young and the old were its victims. On the first symptom the patients fell into a profound melancholy and seemed to abandon all hope of recovery. This moral prostration aggravated their physical condition, and mental depression hastened the time of death. The fear of contagion was so great that but few persons attended the sick.

The clergy, encouraged by the Pope, visited the bedsides of the dying who bequeathed all their wealth to the Church. The plague was considered on all sides as a punishment inflicted by God, and it was this idea that induced armies of penitents to assemble on the public streets to do penance for their sins. Men and women went half naked along the highways flagellating each other with whips, and, growing desperate with the fall of night, they committed scandalous crimes. In certain places the Jews were accused of being the authors of the plague by poisoning the wells; hence the Hebrews were persecuted, sometimes burned alive by the fanatical sects known as Flagellants, Begardes and Turlupins, who were encouraged in their acts of violence by the priests, notwithstanding the intervention of Clement VI.

Physicians were not only convinced of the contagious nature of the disease, but also believed that it could be transmitted by look and word of mouth. Such doctors obliged their patients to cover their eyes and mouth with a piece of cloth whenever the priest or physician visited the bedside. *"Cum igitur medicus vel sacerdos, vel amicus aliquem infirmum visitare voluerit, moneat et introducat aegrum suos claudere et linteamine operire."*

Guillaume de Machant, poet and *valet de chambre* of Philip the Beautiful, mentions this fact in one of his poems, *i. e.*:

"They did not dare, in the open air

To even speak by stealth,

Lest each one's breath might carry death

By poisoning the other's health."

And, in the preface of the "Decameron," Boccaccio remarks in his turn, "The plague communicated direct, as fire to combustible matter. They were often attacked from simply touching the sick, indeed it was not even necessary to touch them. The danger was the same when you listened to their words or even if they gazed at you."

One thing is certain, that is, that those who nursed the patients surely contracted the disease.

All the authorities of the Middle Ages concur in their statements as to the contagious nature of the plague. The rules and regulations enforced against the afflicted were barbarous and inhuman. "Persons sick and well, of one family, when the pest developed," says Black,[14] "were held, without distinction, in close confinement in their home, while on the house door a red cross was traced, bearing the sad and desperate epitaph, *'Dieu ayez pitie de nous!'* No one was permitted to leave or enter the plague-stricken house save the physician and nurse, or other persons who might be authorized by the Government. The doors of such dwellings were guarded and kept closed until such a time as the imprisoned had all died or recovered their health."

We can well judge of the terror inspired by the pestilence by the precautions taken by the physicians in attendance on the sick. In his treatise on the plague

Mauget describes the costume worn by those who approached the bedsides of patients:

"The costumes worn, says he, "were of Levant morocco, the mask having crystal eyes and a long nose filled with subtile perfumes. This nose was in the form of a snout, with the openings one on each side; these openings served for respiratory passages and were well filled at the anterior portion with drugs, so that at each breath they contained a medicated air. Under a cloak the doctor also wore buskins made of morocco; closely sewed breeches were attached to the bottines above the ankle; the shirt, the hat and gloves were also of soft morocco."

Thus accoutered the doctor resembled a modern diver clad in a bathing suit of leather.

In order not to alarm the population all public references to funerals were forbidden. In the ordinances of magistrates of Paris, passed September 13, 1553, we read, "And likewise be it declared that the aforesaid Chamber forbids by statute all criers of funerals and wines, and all others, no matter what be their state or condition, to render for sale at any church, house, doorway or gate of this city, or on the streets thereof, any black cloth or mourning stuffs such as are used for mortuary purposes, under penalty of forfeiture of their licenses and property, and confiscation of all goods, especially of the aforesaid black cloths."

Let it be well understood that the great epidemics of plague in the sixth and twelfth centuries were of a nature to terrify ignorant populations. The narratives of the historians of that epoch show them to be imbued with the superstitious ideas of antiquity. This attack of an invisible enemy whose blows fell right and left paralyzed and terrified every one. "In the midst of this orgie of death," remarks Anglada, "the thought of self-preservation absorbed every other sentiment. Dominated by this selfish instinct the human mind shamelessly displayed its cowardice, egotism and superstition. Social ties were rudely sundered, the affections of the heart laid aside. The sick were deserted by their relatives; all flew with horror from the plague-breathing air and contact with the dreadful disease. The corpses of the victims of the epidemic abandoned without sepulture exhaled a horrible putrid odor, and became the starting point of new infectious centres. The worse disorder overthrew all conditions of existence. Human passion raged uncontrolled; the voice of authority was no longer respected; the wheels of civilization ceased to revolve."

As to the other epidemics of the plague that periodically devastated France from the fourteenth to the eighteenth century we possess but few historical documents. We have had in our hands an opuscule by Pierre Sordes, who was attacked by the plague in 1587, at the age of twenty, who afterward wrote a treatise on the epidemic, which work he dedicated to Cardinal de Sourdis, the Archbishop of Aquitaine.

The author in this monograph endeavors to explain the remedies then in use for preservation against the infection of the disease. "Avoid all fatigue, anger, intemperance, too much association with women, as the act ennervates our forces and enfeebles our spirits. One should clothe himself in the wools of Auvergne and the camulets of Escot." Moreover, says our author, "one should perfume his clothes with laurel, rosemary, serpolet, marjolane, sage, fennel, sweetbriar, myrrh, and frankincense." When the room was to be disinfected "one should use fumigations of good dry hay. One should not go out early without eating and taking a drink. One should close the ears with a little cotton scented with musk and hold in his mouth a clove or piece of angelica root. One should hold in his hand a piece of sponge saturated in vinegar, which should be smelled frequently. One should wear upon his stomach an acorn filled with quicksilver and a small pouch containing arsenic. Finally, one should take twice a week a pill composed of aloes, myrrh, and saffron."

Notwithstanding all these precautions, Pierre Sordes was attacked by the plague; having a buboe in the left groin, which caused him acute pain and to which he applied "*un emplastre de diachyllum cum gummis*" and afterwards a blister. Not being able to obtain resolution, feeling his strength undermined and perceiving his entire body "covered with black lumps and spots, fatal prognostic signs to all who are found thus marked, I called for a surgeon, the last one left alive, and he brought his cautery and with it pierced through the apostume. From then the fever disappeared little by little, and I was perfectly cured eight days after the application of the aforesaid cautery, with the exception that, reading in a draught Bartas "Treatise on the Plague," I brought on another attack of fever that well nigh carried me off.

"This is my experience at Figeac in the year 1587, when the plague destroyed 2500 people, with all the miseries and calamities that can be read in Greek and Roman histories."

LE MAL DES ARDENTS.

Towards the end of the tenth century a new epidemic appeared in Europe, the ravages of which spread terror among the people of the Occident; this disease was known by the name of *mal des ardents*, sacred fire, St. Anthony's fire, St. Marcell's fire, and hell fire.

This great epidemic of the Middle Ages is considered by many modern writers as one of the forms of ergotism, notwithstanding the contrary conclusions arrived at by the Commission of 1776, composed of such men as Jussieu, Paulet, Saillant, and Teissier, who were ordered to report as to the nature of the disease by the Royal Society. According to the work of this Commission the *mal des ardents* was a variety of plague, with buboes, carbuncles and petechial spots, while St. Anthony's fire was only gangrenous ergotism. This is a remarkable example of the confusion into which scientific facts were allowed to fall through the fault of careless authors. It is in such instances that we may estimate the importance of history. We find in the "Chronicles of Frodoard," in the year 945, the following: "The year 945, in the history of Paris and its numerous suburban villages, a disease called *ignis plaga* attacked the limbs of many persons, and consumed them entirely, so that death soon finished their sufferings. Some few survived, thanks be to the intercession of the Saints; and even a considerable number were cured in the Church of Notre Dame de Paris. Some of these, believing themselves out of danger, left the church; but the fires of the plague were soon relighted, and they were only saved by returning to Notre Dame."

Sauvel, the translator of Frodoard, remarks that at this epoch the Church of Notre Dame served as a hospital for the sick attacked by the epidemic, and sometimes contained as high as six hundred patients.

Another historian of the time was Raoul Glaber,[15] who mentions that "in 993 a murderous malady prevailed among men. This was a sort of hidden fire, *ignis occultus*, the which attacked the limbs and detached them from the trunk after having consumed the members. Among some the devouring effect of this fire took place in a single night.

"In 1039," continues our author, "divine vengeance again descended on the human race with fearful effect and destroyed many inhabitants of the world, striking alike the rich and the poor, the aristocrat and the peasant. Many persons lost their limbs and dragged themselves around as an example to those who came after them."

In the *Chronicle of France*, from the commencement of the Monarchy up to 1029,[16] the monk Adhemar speaks of the epidemic in the following terms: "In these times a pestilential fire (*pestilential ignis*) attacked the population of Limousin; an infinite number of persons of both sexes were consumed by an invisible fire."

Michael Felibien, a Benedictine friar of Saint Maur, also left notes on the epidemic of gangrene. He states in his *History of Paris*: "In the same year, 1129, Paris, as the rest of France, was afflicted by the *maladie des ardents*. This disease, although known from the mortality it caused in the years 945 and 1041, was all the more terrible inasmuch as it appeared to have no remedy. The mass of blood, already corrupted by internal heat which devoured the entire body, pushed its fluids outwards into tumors, which degenerated into incurable ulcers and thus killed off thousands of people."

We could make many more citations, derived from ancient writers, but we think we have quoted enough authors to prove that the *mal des ardents* was only the plague confounded with the symptoms known as gangrenous ergotism. Could it not have been a plague of a gangrenous type? We cannot positively affirm, however, that it had no connection with poisoning by the *sphacelia* developed in grain, particularly on rye. Its onset was sudden, and often very rapidly followed by a fatal termination. The *mal des ardents* had no prodroma with general symptoms and marked periods, as in gangrenous ergotism, but it had, to the contrary, an irregular march, rapid in its evolution, "devouring," as Mezeray says, "the feet, the arms, the face, and private parts, commencing most generally in the groin."

THE ERUPTIVE FEVERS OF THE SIXTH CENTURY —— VARIOLA, MEASLES, SCARLATINA.

Before the sixth century, the terrible period of the plague, one never heard of the eruptive fevers. Small-pox, measles and scarlet fever were unknown to the ancients. Neither Hippocrates nor Galen nor any of the Greek physicians who practiced in Rome make mention of these diseases. The historians and poets of Greece and Italy who have written largely on medical subjects remain mute on these three great questions in pathology. Some authors have endeavored to torture texts for the purpose of throwing light on the contagious exanthemata, but they have not been repaid for their fresh imagination.[17] It is admitted to-day that the eruptive fevers are comparatively new diseases, which made their appearance in the Middle Ages.

The first document that the history of medicine possesses on this point is that left by Marius, Bishop of Aventicum, in Switzerland, who says, in his chronicle, "*Anno 570, morbus validus cum profluvio ventris et variola, Italiam Galliamque valde affecit.*"[18]

Ten years later, Gregory of Tours described the symptoms of the new disease in the following terms:[19]

"The fifth year of the reign of Childebert, 580, the region of Auvergne was inundated by a flood and numerous weather disasters, which were followed by a terrible epidemic that invaded the whole of Gaul. Those attacked had violent fevers, accompanied by vomiting, great pain in the neighborhood of the kidneys, and a heaviness in the head and neck. Matter rejected by the stomach looked yellowish and even green, many deeming this to be some secret poison. The peasants called the pustules corals.[20] Sometimes, after the application of cups to the shoulders or limbs, blisters were raised, which, when broken, gave issue to sanious matter, which oftentimes saved the patient. Drinks composed of simples to combat the effects of the poison were also very efficacious.

"This disease, which commenced in the month of August, attacked all the very young children and carried them off.

"In those days Chilperic was also seriously afflicted, and as the King commenced to convalesce his youngest son was taken with the malady, and when his extremity was perceived he was given baptism. Shortly afterwards he was better, and his eldest brother, named Chlodobert, was attacked in his turn. They placed the Prince in a litter and carried him to Soissons, in the chapel of Saint Medard; there he was placed in contact with the good Saint's tomb, and made vows to him for recovery, but, very weak and almost without breath, he rendered his soul to God in the middle of night.

"In those days, Austrechilde, wife of King Gontran, also died of the disease; while Nantin, Count of Angouleme, also succumbed to the same malady, his body becoming so black that it appeared as though calcined charcoal."

Gregory of Tours, in another chapter, narrates:

"The year of the reign of King Childebert, 582, another epidemic broke out; this was accompanied by blackish spots of a malignant nature, with pustules and vesicles, and carried off many victims.

"Touraine was cruelly devastated by this disease. The patient attacked by fever soon had the surface of his body covered by vesicles and small pustules. The vesicles were white and very hard, presenting no element of softness, and were accompanied by great pain; when they had attained maturity they broke and allowed the humor within to escape. Their sticking to the clothing of the body added considerably to the pain. Medical art was wholly impotent in the presence of this malady, at least when God did not come to the doctor's aid.

"The wife of Count Eborin, who was attacked by the disease, was so covered by vesicles that neither her hand nor the sole of her foot nor any portion of her body was exempt; even her eyes remained closed. Soon after the fever ceased the fall of the pustules occurred, and the patient recovered without more inconvenience."

Small-pox came, then, from the Orient—that eternal center of all pestilences and curses. From the seventh century the Saracen armies spread the malady wherever they passed—in Syria, Egypt, and Spain; in their turn, the Crusaders, in returning from the Holy Land, brought the disease into France, England, and Germany. From thence the great epidemics of the twelfth and thirteenth centuries, after which the small-pox became epidemic, appearing and disappearing without causation, but always destroying myriads of victims. "In 1445," says Sauvel "from the month of August to Saint Andres' day (November 30), over 6,000 infants died in Paris from small-pox.[21] The physicians knew neither the nature nor the treatment of the new disease.[22]

The measles was first noted at the same time as the small-pox, making its first appearance as an epidemic in the sixth century.

It is more than probable that the measles originated in Egypt, and according to Borsieri, it had such an extension throughout Western Europe that there were but few persons who had not suffered attacks. The history of measles, however, is less clearly defined than that of small-pox, although Anglada says that it figured among the *spotted diseases*, of which Gregory of Tours speaks.[23] But it was only in the sixteenth century that Prosper Martian exactly describes the disease.

Says Martian, "It is a disease of a special type peculiar to children, who can no more avoid it than small pox. It commences with a violent fever, followed, towards the third day, by an eruption of small red spots, which become elevated by degrees, making the skin feel rough to the touch. The fever lasts until the fifth day, and when it has ceased the papules commence to disappear."

Measles was designated in the middle ages under the name *Morbilli*, which signified a petty plague, the same that *Morbus* meant a special plague. It is then fair to presume that the type of disease was no more serious than it is at the present day.

It is probable that the measles of the sixth century included at the same time small-pox, measles and scarlet fever, of which the ancients made no differential diagnosis. Anglada affirms the co-existence of all forms of eruptive fevers and gives the following reasons:

"The contemporaneous appearance of variola and rubeola represents the first manifestation of an epidemic constitution, resulting from a collection of unknown influences as to their nature, but manifest by their effects. The earth was from thence prepared to receive scarlatina, and it soon came to bear its baleful fruits. We do meet some mention of scarlet fever in the writings of the Arabian School, but it is merely suspected and only vaguely indicated. But when we remember how difficult it often is to diagnose at first between variola and measles, we are not astonished at the indecision manifested in adding another exanthematous affection to the medical incognito. It was only after innumerable observations and the experience of several centuries that the third new disease received its nosological baptism. There is nothing to prove that it did not co-operate with earlier epidemics of variola and rubeola, remaining undistinguished as to type, however."

What clearly proves that there was confusion between the various fevers of exanthemata is that Ingrassias describes scarlatina in 1510, under the name of *rosallia*, adding, "Some think the measles and *rosallia* are the same malady; as for me, I have determined their differences on many occasions. *Nonnulli sunt qui morbillos idem cum rossalia esse existimant. Nos autem soepissime distinctos esse affectus, nostrismet oculis, non aliorum duntaxat relationi confidentes inspeximus."*[24]

These facts appear conclusive enough to admit that measles and scarlet fever are, like variola, the products of the epidemic constitution developed during the sixth century, as contemporaries of the bubonic plague, all these maladies representing the medical constitution of the first centuries of the Middle Age.

THE SWEATING SICKNESS OF ENGLAND.

The name of Sweating Sickness was given to the great epidemic of fever that appeared in England in the fifteenth century, and from thence extended over Continental Europe. This epidemic broke out in the month of September, 1486, in the army of Henry VII., encamped in Wales, and soon reached London, extending over the British Isles with frightful rapidity. Its appearance was alarming and during its duration, which was only a month, it made a considerable number of victims. "It was so terrible and so acute that within the memory of man none had seen its like."

This epidemic reappeared in England in 1513, 1517 and 1551. It was preceded by very moist weather and violent winds. The mortality was great, patients often dying in the space of two hours; in some instances half the population of a town being carried off. The epidemic of 1529 can only be called murderous; King Henry VIII. was attacked and narrowly escaped death. Although flying from village to village the nobility of England paid an enormous tribute to the King of Terrors. The Ambassador from France to London, M. du Bellay, writing on the 21st of July, 1529, remarks, "The day I visited the Bishop of Canterbury eighteen of the household died in a few hours. I was about the only one left to tell the tale, and am far from recovered yet."

This same year the sweating sickness spread all over Europe. It made terrible ravages in Holland, Germany and Poland. At the famous synod of Luther and Zwingle, held at Marburg, the Reformed ministers seized by fear of death prayed for relief from the pestilence. At Augsburg in three months eighteen thousand people were attacked and fourteen hundred died.

This epidemic did not extend as far as Paris, but it developed in the north of France and Belgium. Mezeray mentions this fact in the following terms: "A certain disease appeared this year (1529), commencing in England. It was of a contagious nature, and passed over from France to the Lower Countries, and thus spread over most of Europe. Those attacked sweated profusely; it was for this reason that the malady was called the *English Sweat.* First one had a hard chill, then a very high fever, which carried the patient off in twenty-four hours, unless promptly remedied."

Fernel, physician to Henry II., who practiced in Paris, likewise speaks of this sudorific sickness in one of his works.[25] He says: *"Febres sudorificae quae insolentes magno terrore in omnem inferiorem Germaniam, in Galliam, Belgicam, et in Britanniam ab anno Christi millesimo quingentesimo vigesim autumno potissimum pervagatae sunt."*

It prevailed almost always in summer and autumn, especially when the weather was moist and foggy. Contrary to what is seen in other epidemics, it was observed that the weak and poor, the old and infants were not attacked as often as robust persons and those in affluent circumstances.

The symptoms noted by physicians, such as Kaye and Bacon, may be classed into three distinct periods: 1. The period of chill, characterized by pains and formication in the limbs an extraordinary prostration of the physical forces—a tremulous, shaky period. 2. The period of sweat, preceded by a burning heat all over the body and an unquenchable feverish thirst. The patient was agitated, disquieted by terror and despair. Many complained of spasms in the stomach, followed sometimes by nausea and vomiting, suffocation and lumbar pains—a constant symptom ever—headache, with palpitation of the heart and præcordial anxiety. 3. This period was announced by a high delirium, sometimes muttering, sometimes loquacious; a fetid sweaty odor, irregular pulse, coma, and, in the last-named condition, death always occurred.

The duration of the disease was most frequently but a few hours, rarely exceeding a day, whether the termination was favorable or fatal.

Convalescence was always long, often being complicated by diarrhœa or dropsy. It has been remarked in this connection that the malady might be confounded with the miliary sweat observed in Picardy and central France, but in the first named disease no cutaneous eruption was observed. Fernel clearly affirms this statement, as he says: "In this affection there is no carbuncle, bubo, exanthema nor eczema, but simply a hypersecretion of sweat."

Such was the sweating sickness of the sixteenth century, which made so few victims in France, but which destroyed so many people in England and Germany. The origin of this disease has been often discussed, and also its nature; but all theories emitted by various authors partake of the doctrines of other days and are too antiquated to be revamped. We will content ourselves with saying that the classification of periods made by us is logical, and we consider the sweating sickness of the fifteenth century as a pernicious fever, in which the sweating stage predominated and consequently became the characteristic symptom of the affection.

THE SCURVY.

It has been supposed by many that Hippocrates described scurvy under the name of *enlarged spleen*, an affection attributed to the use of stagnant water and characterized by tumefaction of the gums, foul breath, pale face, and ulceration of the lower limbs. But the study of this Hippocratic passage leads us to think that these symptoms were more of the character of scrofula than of scurvy. The recital by Pliny of the diseases of the Roman soldiers while on an expedition to Germany seems to indicate scurvy, which Coelius Aurelianus, and after him the Arabian physicians, claims presented only a slight analogy to that affection.

Springer thinks that we may find the first traces of scurvy in the expedition of the Normans to Wineland, in the first years of the eleventh century. In admitting that the men commanded by Eric Thorstein were obliged to winter on the western shores of Wineland and almost all succumbed to an endemic malady of that country, proves that it was nothing but scurvy, although that word's only signification, in Danish, is ulceration of the mouth.

We have, besides, another document, which has great authentic value, a proof transmitted to us by our earliest and best chronicler of the Middle Ages, by Joinville, the friend and companion of Saint Louis in his Crusade into Palestine. In his memoirs he gives a very succinct recital of the epidemic of famine and scurvy which attacked the French army on the banks of the Nile in 1248, just after the battles of Mansourah. Says Joinville: "After the two battles just mentioned, commenced our great miseries in the army; at the end of nine days the bodies of our dead soldiers arose to the surface of the water (their tissues were corrupted and rotten), and these corpses floated to a point between our two camps (those of the King and the Duke of Bourgogne), at a point where a bridge touched the water. So many had been slain that a great crowd of corpses floated on the stream for a long distance. The bodies of the dead Saracens were sickening; the army servants threw open a portion of the bridge and permitted the dead infidels to float down the river, but they buried the dead Crusaders in great pits dug in the ground. I saw among other dead the body of the Chamberlain of the Count D'Artois, and many other friends among the slain.

"The only fish we had eaten for four months were of the variety called *barbus*, and these *barbus* fed on the dead bodies, and for this cause and other miseries of the country where never a drop of rain fell sickness entered our army of such a sort that the flesh on the limbs dried and the skin on the legs became black and like old leather boots, and many sick rotted in their groin; and all having the last named symptom died. Another sign of death was when the nose bled."

The relation of Joinville leaves no doubt as to the nature of the epidemic that attacked the Crusaders. Here we have a pen picture of the debility, the hemorrhages, the livid ecchymosis of the skin, the fungous tumefaction and bleeding of the gums, which characterize the disease known as scurvy.

According to the writings of some German physicians of the fifteenth century, this malady was endemic in the septentrional portions of Europe upon the shores of the Baltic Sea. In Holland numerous epidemics of scurvy were observed among the lower classes of the population, coinciding with bad conditions of public hygiene. Food consisting of salt and smoked meats, dwellings located on marshy ground, cold atmospheres charged with fogs, etc., etc.

This was the same affection that attacked our colonies in Canada, but at that time we had no knowledge of the therapeutic indications in such emergencies, and quote as a proof of this a remarkable observation inscribed on the registers of Cartier on his vessels during his sojourn in Canada: "The disease commenced in our midst in a curious and unknown manner; some patients lost their flesh and their limbs grew black and swollen like charcoal, and some were covered over with bloody splotches like purpura; after which the disease showed itself on the hips, thighs, arms, and neck, and in all the mouth was infected and rotten at the gums, so that all the flesh fell off to the roots of the teeth, which also most often dropped out; and so terrible was this plague that on my three ships by February only ten healthy men were about out of a crew of over a hundred.

"And, as the disease was unknown to us, the Captain of the ships was asked to open a few bodies to see if we could possibly detect the lesion and thus be able to protect the survivors. We found the hearts of the dead to be white and withered, surrounded by a rose colored effusion; the liver healthy, but the lung black and mortified and all its blood retired to the sac of the heart. The spleen likewise was impaired for about two finger-lengths as though rubbed by a rough stone."

From this autopsy rudely made[26] it is true we discern most of the signs of scrofula; a profound alteration of the blood and an effusion of the liquids into certain viscera, denoting a diminution in the amount of fibrin and the number of globules, alterations that also serve to explain the tendency to hemorrhages observed in very serious cases of scurvy.

LEPROSY.

Leprosy is a disease originating in the Orient; Egypt and Judea were formerly the principal infected centers. It was the return of an expedition to Palestine, under Pompey, that imported the malady to Italy. In the first years of the Christian Era it is mentioned by Celsus, who advised that it should be treated by sweating, aided by vapor baths. Some years later Areteus used hellebore, sulphur baths, and the flesh of vipers taken as food, a treatment adopted by others, as, for instance, Musa and Archigenes.

In the second century the disease was in Gaul; Soranus treated the lepers of Aquitaine, who were numerous.[27]

According to Velly, leprosy was common in France in the middle of the eighth century epoch, when Nicholas, Abbot of Corbeil, constructed a leper hospital, which was never much frequented until after the Crusades of the eleventh and fourteenth centuries. At this period the number of lepers, or *ladres*, a name given to the unfortunates in remembrance of their patron saint, St. Lazarus, became so great that every town and village was obliged to build a leper house in order to isolate the afflicted. Under Louis VIII. there were 2,000 of these hospitals; later the number of such asylums reached 19,000.

According to the historians of this time, when a man was suspected to be a leper he could have no social relations without making full declaration as to what the real nature of his complaint might be. Without this precaution his acts were void, from the capitulary of Pepin, which dissolved all marriage contracts with lepers, to the law of Charlemagne, that forbade their associating with healthy persons. The fear of contagion was such that in places where no leprosy existed they built small houses for any one who might be attacked; these houses were called *bordes*.[28] A gray mantle, a hat and wallet, were also supplied the victims, also a *tartarelle*, a species of rattle, or a small bell, with which they warned all passers near not to approach. They also had a cup placed on the far side of the road, in which all persons might drop alms without going near the leper.

Leper houses were enriched, little by little, by the liberality of kings and nobles and the people, and to be a leper became less inhuman and horrible than at the beginning.

Lepers, however, were forced to submit to severe police regulations. They were forbidden under the severest penalties from having sexual relations with healthy persons, for such intimacy was considered as the most dangerous method of conveying the contagion. After entering a leper house the victim was considered as dead under the civil law, and in order to make the patients better understand their position the clergy accompanied them to their asylum, the same as to their funeral, throwing the cemetery dust on them while saying: "Enter into no house save your asylum. When you speak to an outsider stand to the windward. When you ask alms sound your rattle. You must not go far from the asylum without your leper's robe. You must drink from no well or spring save on your own grounds. You must pass no plates nor cups without first putting on your gloves. You must not go barefooted, nor walk in narrow streets, nor lean against walls, trees, or doors, nor sleep on the edge of the road," etc.

When dead they were interred in the lepers' cemetery by their fellow-sufferers.

Separated from society, these pariahs, living together, sometimes reproduced their own species, and finished their days in the most frightful cachexia, awaking only contempt, disgust, and repulsion among the healthy of the outside world.

It is true that each time that sanitary measures were relaxed by the authorities—such, for instance, as the perfect isolation of the patients—an increase in the number of lepers was noticeable. When this was observed the old-time ordinances were enforced again with vigor. It was thus in 1371 the Provost of Paris issued an edict enjoining all lepers to leave the Capital within fifteen days, under heavy corporal and pecuniary penalties; and in 1388, all lepers were forbidden to enter Paris without special permission; in 1402 this restriction was renewed, "under penalty of being taken by the executioner and his deputies and detained for a month on a diet of bread and water, and afterwards perpetual banishment from the kingdom." Finally, in April, 1488, it was announced "all persons attacked by that abominable, very dangerous and contagious malady known as leprosy, must leave Paris before Easter and retire to their hospitals from the date of issuance of this edict, under penalty of imprisonment for a month on bread and water; and, where they had property, the sequestration of their houses and jewels and arbitrary corporal punishment; it was permitted them, however, to send things to them by servants, the latter being in health."

We can understand from this how these poor wretches, at different epochs, were accused of horrible crimes, among other things poisoning rivers, wells, and fountains. As regards this accusation, says the author of the *Dictionnaire des Mœurs des Francais*, Philip le Long burned a certain number of these poor devils at the stake and confiscated their wealth, giving it to the Order of Malta and St. Lazare.

The historians and chronicalers of the eleventh and twelfth century often designated the person attacked by leprosy by the name of *mesel, mezel, meseau* or *mesiaus.* Meantime Barbazin pretends that it is necessary to make a distinction.[29]

Mesel, according to Barbazin, was a person covered with sores and ulcers, while the leper was an insensible man. He thinks that *mesellerie* was at its origin a different affection than leprosy, and that these two diseases have been wrongly confounded. "They have both served," says he, "to designate a frightful disease, that is reputed the most dangerous of all maladies."

As supporting this assertion of Barbazin, we have found in the Romanesque tongue some documents strongly confirming this point. They appear more interesting, inasmuch as they have heretofore been unknown to medical literature, as, for instance:

"Seneschal, I now demand of you, said he (Saint Louis), which you love better, whether you be *mesiaus*, or whether you commit a mortal sin; and I, who never have lied, responded that rather would I commit thirty mortal sins than be *mesiaus*." (Joinville, *Histoire de Saint Louis*.)

The leprosy, however, was not an absolute cause for divorce, as we note in the following passage: "A man can leave his wife only for fornication, and not alone for leprosy, and lepers may marry; and one may cancel marriage if the husband become leper, and the same may be said of the bride."

In the same manuscript another analogous fact shows the invalidation of the marital act for the reason of *mesellerie* complicated by impotence or barrenness.

"A woman who through impotence has lost that which is necessary to her, so that he cannot cohabit with her, for the reason that he is *mesiaus*, may marry another, telling the latter, however, that the first she married was worth nothing, not even an infant, as he could not cohabit; that nothing can prevent cohabitation in marriage nor the begetting of children."

Individuals attacked by *mesellerie* were in reality outside the pale of the law. For we read in fact in the *"Coutume de Beauvoisis,* cap. 39," that *"mesiaus* must not be called on as witnesses, for custom accords them no place in the conversation of gentlemen."

"The second reason is that when a *mesiaus* calls on a healthy man, or when a healthy man calls on a *mesel*, the *mesiaus* may put in the defense that he is beyond the reach of worldly law, and cannot be held responsible in such a case."

These unfortunates besides could not inherit nor dispose of their own wealth during their lives. The following passage from the "ancient customs of Normandy" bears witness, *i. e.*:

"The *mesel* can be no man's heir from the time his disease is developed, but he may have a life interest, as though he were not a *mesel*."

The same as in many other diseases the leprosy presented itself under different forms and various degrees of gravity, as is proved from the following passage from *Le Pelerinage de l'humaine lignee:*

"Homs, qui ne scet bien discerner

Entre sante et maladie,

Entre le grant mesellerie

Entre le moienne et le meure."

This gravity of different forms of leprosy has likewise been mentioned by the Arabian school, and notably by Avicenna, who had seen numerous cases complicated with ulcerations of the genital organs; also, by the Englishman, Gilbert, who wrote in the thirteenth century regarding the existence of several species of leprosy, which could not always be easily distinguished by reason of the uncertainty of their symptoms. As to its character as a constitutional malady we have the word of the Syrian Jaliah ebn Serapion, who attributes its connection to the predominance of certain humors; finally, Valescus of Tarentum insists on the heredity of the disease.

The leprosy, the pork measles and the *mesellerie* were then only clinical forms of a single affection of a contagious nature—a hereditary disease whose symptoms appeared successively on the skin, in the mucous membranes, the viscera and in the nervous system. It then required a diathesis, which resembled greatly in its evolution that of syphilis, with which it has often been confounded.

The physicians of leper hospitals have left behind a great number of medical documents bearing on the characteristics of the disease, but their observations are so confused that we can only conclude that they considered all cutaneous maladies as belonging to the same constitutional vice.

They recognized, however, the *ladrerrie* (disease arising from measly pork), by the following symptoms, the same being laid down by Guy de Chauliac:

"Eyelids and eyebrows swollen, falling of eye-lashes and eyebrows, which are replaced by a finer quality of hair; ulceration of septum of the nose, odor of ozoena, granulated tongue, fœtid breath, painful breathing, thickening and hardness of the lips, with fissures and lividity of same; gums tumefied and ulcerated; furfuraceous scales in the hair, purple face, fixed expression, hideous aspect; forehead smooth and shiny like a horn; pustules on face; veins on chest much developed; breasts hard."

"Thinness of muscles of the hand, especially thumb and index finger; lividity and cracking of the nails; coldness of the extremities; presence of a serpiginous eruption; insensibility of the legs, collections of nodosities around the joints; under the influence of cold elevations appeared on the cutis, making it appear like goose-skin."

"Sensation of pricking, ulcerations of skin; sleep uneasy, fetidity of sweat; feeble pulse, bad odor of blood, which is viscid and oily to the touch and gritty after incineration, likewise of a violet black color."

The contagious characteristic of leprosy through sexual relation was noticed by physicians attached to hospitals, and was the subject of police restriction by public sanitary officers. Thus in the thirteenth century the celebrated Roger Bacon, surnamed the admirable doctor, wrote that commerce with a leprous woman could be followed by very serious consequences. This opinion was corroborated by a physician of the University of Oxford, his contemporary John of Gaddsen, and by the observations of Bernard Gordon, a celebrated practitioner of Montpellier. We all know the history of a Countess who came to be treated for leprosy at Montpellier, when a Bachelor in Medicine charged with the task of dressing her sores, fell desperately in love with the leper lady, and from his *amours* contracted most serious cutaneous disease.

At this period the leprosy had already begun to assume a venereal type of marked character, and many prostitutes suffered from attacks. As we all are aware, Jean Manardi, an Italian doctor, has fully expressed his opinion on this subject. In a letter addressed to a friend, Michel Santana, one of the first specialists who treated pox, Manardi remarks: "This disease has attacked Valencia, in Spain, being spread broadcast by a famous courtesan, who, for the price of fifty crowns, accorded her favors to a nobleman suffering from leprosy. This woman having been tainted, in her turn contaminated all the young men who called on her, so that more than four hundred were affected in a brief space of time. Some of these, having followed the fortunes of King Charles into Italy, carried and spread this cruel malady in their track."

Another Italian physician, Andre Mathiole, likewise shows the identity of leprosy with syphilis,—in the following terms: "Some authors have written that the French have taken this disease from impure commerce with leprous women while traversing the mountains of Italy."[30]

We could easily multiply such citations to complete the facts observed by Fernel and Ambroise Pare in France, and also by many Italian physicians, from whence it would be easy to understand why Manardi came to the following conclusion: "Those who have connection with a woman who has had recent *amours* with a leper, a courtesan in whose womb the seeds of disease may linger, sometimes contract leprosy and at other times suffer from other maladies of a more or less serious nature, according to their predispositions."

This modification from *measles* (the disease from corrupt pork diet) into leprosy of the venereal type is made progressively through the intermediary of the ordinary agencies of prostitution,—bawds and libertines,—who for a very long period eluded the wise laws ordained by sanitary police for the restriction of lepers. In 1543, the affection was so wide-spread as to be beyond sanitary control, and the edict of Francois I., re establishing leper hospitals, amounted to nothing. There were too many poxed people. The Hospital of Lourcine, which was specially devoted to these cases at Paris contained 600 patients in 1540, and in the wards of Trinity Hospital and the Hotel Dieu there were many more. It was the same in the Provinces, notably at Tolouse, which had the merit of creating the first venereal hospital ever instituted, under the Gascon name of "*Houspital das rognousez de la rougno de Naples.*" Finally, fifty years later, in 1606, for want of lepers, the leper asylums were officially closed. Henry IV., in a proclamation, gave those remaining "to poor gentlemen and crippled soldiers."

Thus ended the epidemic of leprosy in France, which had prevailed from the second century, observing the same progress in other countries of Western Europe during the same period of time. Syphilis, the product of the venereal maladies of antiquity and the leprosy of the Middle Ages, announced a new era; syphilis was thus contemporaneous with the *Renaissance.*

In the collection of Guy Patin's letters, there is an interesting document relating to the connection of leprosy and syphilis, as witness the principal passage:

"It was not long since that I saw in Auvergne a patient who was suspected of measles (*hog disease*), for the reason that his family had the reputation of being thus afflicted, though he bore on his body no marks of the disease. This led me to recall the fact that some families in Paris have been suspected of this taint; but really we have no measles or leprosy here. In former times there was a hospital dedicated to such cases in the Faubourg Saint Denis. I have noticed no cases in Champagne, Normandy nor Picardy, although in all these Provinces I found asylums formerly used for such cases that are now turned into hospitals for plague victims. In former times leprosy was confounded with pox, through the ignorance of doctors and the barbarity of the age; nevertheless, there are yet a few lepers in Provence, Languedoc and Poitou."

We have here the authority of Guy Patin for saying that leprosy had almost entirely disappeared from France in the sixteenth century.

Although modern Faculties are prone to insist that the real science of medicine only dates back its origin to the discovery of the microscope, and that the study of antique medicine is only a retrospective exposition calculated to show the slight scientific value of ancient observations, I assert that the many observations recorded by our medical ancestors are of immense value. Let us cite, as a single instance, this transformation of a constitutional malady, attenuated by time, transmitted by heredity through the same masses of people for ten centuries,—populations having a similar diathesis,—a disease taking a new vigor and attacking other generations, but destined in a given time to disappear, most probably, in its turn, in another unknown metamorphosis. Such an idea may cause a smile in that haughty *section hors rang* in medicine, which is so devoted to the culture of specific germs that but one idea can certainly be adopted as an irrefutable dogma in medicine—that is, if the facts it represents coincide with the modifications of the wag—in the tail end of a bacillus.

As for myself, I remain convinced that everything seen in modern times, through the objective even of an instrument of precision, cannot destroy the accumulated work of twenty centuries of medical observation and study.

Scientiæ enim per additamenta fiunt.

THE SYPHILIS.

If the true syphilis—the variety that appeared in the fifteenth century—was unknown in the Middle Ages, there still exist documents which fully affirm the existence of contagious venereal diseases several hundreds of years before the Italian wars of Charles VIII. and Louis XII. The maladies which, in times of antiquity, afflicted the Hebrews and Romans, as a result of impure sexual commerce, are to-day only the results of the progress made by prostitution after the Crusades; that is to say, they are merely the products of debauchery and leprous virus imported from the Orient.

As early as the twelfth century France knew the *mal malin* or *mal boubil,* an affection characterized by sores and ulcerations on the arms and genital organs. Gauthier de Coinci, Prior of the Abbey of St. Medard de Soissons, at the beginning of the thirteenth century considered these maladies as impure and contagious, and warned his priests in the following verselets:

"The monk, the church clerk and the priest

Must not defile themselves the least,

But with good conscience and pure heart

Keep their hands off from private part.

Pray God at morning and at night

To hide corruption from their sight;

The *mal boubil* the *mal malan*

Comes ever to each sinning man."

We are permitted to suppose from these lines that the disease was localized in "a wicked place that the hands must not touch," and that it was only an affection of the same nature as the *gorre* and *grand gorre,* one of the numerous expressions applied to all contagious maladies of the sexual organs. This fact cannot be contested, for at the same epoch, in a poem entitled *"Des XXIII*

Manieres de Vilains," we find an imprecation launched by this anonymous author against all blackguards and bawds:

"That they may be

Itchy, poxed, and apostumed,

Covered with ulcers, badly rheumed,

Full of fever, jaundice sapped,

That they may be, also, clapped."

Or, as given in French:

"Qu ils aient ...

Rogne, variole et apostume,

Et si aient plente de grume,

Plente de fievre et de jaunisse,

Et si aient la chade-pisse"

Now, the opuscle, from which these verses are derived, was reprinted in 1833 by Francisque Michel, and is contemporaneous with the manuscripts of the thirteenth century, analyzed by M. Littre in *a note on syphilis,*[31] where our erudite author says: "At this epoch the venereal diseases had an analogous form to those we observe to-day."

This document dates back 200 years before the discovery of America, and is duly authenticated by the testimony of Guillaume Saliceti, a physician and Italian priest of the thirteenth century. "When a man has received a corruption of the penis, after having cohabited with an obscene woman or for other cause, there comes a tumor in the groin."[32] And some years after Lanfranc, a student of Salicetis, wrote, in his turn, in his *Parva Cyrurgia,* that "buboes appear following ulcers on the penis." His description of chancres and other venereal accidents is very remarkable.

Another writer of the thirteenth century, Michel Scott, a Scotch physician, alchemist, and philosopher, who lived in France and Germany for many years, says in one of his numerous works:[33] "Women become livid and have discharges. If a woman is in such a condition and a man cohabit with her his penis is easily diseased, as we often see in adolescents who, ignorant of this fact, often contract a sore organ or are attacked by leprosy. It is also well to know that if a discharge exist at the epoch of conception, the fetus is more or less diseased, and in this case a man must abstain from all connection, and the woman should resist sexual advances, if she have foresight."

This passage leaves no possible doubt as to the existence of blenorrhagia with the discharge and as to the presence of an hereditary syphilitic diathesis, for if the author gives the last-mentioned the name of leprosy it is only for the reason that at this period no positive term was in use to designate venereal diseases,[34] which were confounded with leprosy, with or without reason, the former only being, perhaps, a transformation of the latter.

About a century later, that is to say, on August 8th, 1347, Queen Jeanne of Naples, Countess of Provence, sent to Avignon the statutes relating to the establishment of houses of prostitution in that city. Article IV. of this law regulated police measures in the following terms: "The Queen ordains that every Saturday the bailiff and a barber deputed by the Councilmen shall visit every debauched girl in the place, and if they find any one who has the disease arising from venery, that such a one may be separated from the other girls and lodged apart, to the end that no one may have commerce with her, and that the young may thus avoid contracting disease."[35]

These statutes were first made known by Astruc,[36] and have been inserted without reserve by Grisolle in his *Traite de Pathologie Interne*; also by Cazenave in his *Traite des Syphilides*; but Jules Courtet, and after him Rabutaux and Anglada, have considered these documents as somewhat apocryphal.

We shall not stop to discuss the authenticity of these documents; they have characteristics that make their genuineness almost indisputable. Besides, we can quote other authors against whom no arguments can be used; for instance, we will cite John of Gaddesen, a physician of the English Court, who affirmed that sexual connection with a leprous woman produced ulcers of the penis;[37] besides, his compatriot Gilbert, who described in his *Compendium Medicinal*, in the year 1300, the treatment of gonorrhœa and chancre so common after the Crusades; or Gui du Chauliac, who in 1360 noticed "the ulcers born of commerce with a tainted woman, impure and chancrous (*ex coitu cum fœtida vel immunda vel cancrosa muliere*)."[38] Again, note Torella, of Italy, who considered pox as a contagious malady which had existed from times of antiquity, and which had made its appearance at different epochs, but of which the symptoms, poorly understood by medical men, prevented isolation and its proper pathological identity.[39]

We need not reproduce the text of all the French and especially the Italian doctors, who established the identity of venereal diseases *before the year* 1494— such writers as Montagnana, Petrus Pintor, Nicolas Leonicenus, Joseph Grunpeck, etc. As to these works, they have all been mentioned by Fracastor, in his celebrated *Treatise on Contagious Diseases (de morbis contagiosis)*, a work at once a fine poem, whose Latinity is perfect and a monograph of true scientific exactitude.

Fracastor described the patient as well as the disease: "The victims were sad and broken with pale faces."

"They had chancres on their private parts; these chancres were changeable; when cured at one point they reappeared at another; they always broke out again."

"Pustules with crusts were raised on the skin; in some these commence on the scalp first; this was the usual case; in a few they appeared elsewhere. At first these were small, afterwards increasing in size, appearing like unto the milk crust in children. In some these pustules were small and dry—in others large and humid. Sometimes they were scarlet, sometimes white, sometimes hard and pink. These pustules opened at the end of some days, pouring out an incredible quantity of stinking and nasty liquid, once opened they became true phagedenic ulcers, which not only consumed the flesh but even the bone."

"Those whose upper regions were attacked had malignant fluxions, that eat away the palate, the trachea, the throat and the tonsils. Some patients lost their lips, others their noses, others their eyes, others their private parts."

"Large gummy tumors appeared in many and disfigured the limbs. These growths were often the size of an egg or a French roll of bread. When opened these tumors discharged a whitish mucilaginous liquid. They were principally noted on the arms and legs; while ulcerating sometimes they grew callous, at other times remaining as tumors until death."

"As if this were not sufficient, terrible pains oftimes attacked the limbs; these generally came when the pustules appeared. These pains were long abiding and well nigh insupportable, aching most at night, not only affecting the articulation, hut also the bones and nerves of the limbs. Sometimes the patient had pustules without pains, at other times pains without pustules; but the great majority had pustules and pains."

"The patients were plunged into a condition of languor. They became thin, weak, without appetite, sleeping not, always sad and in a sullen humor, the face and the limbs swollen, with a slight fever at times. Some suffered with pains in the head, pains of long duration, which did not recede before any remedies."

"Although the greater majority of mortals have taken this disease by contagion, it is no less certain that a great number of others contracted it from infection. It is impossible to believe, in fact, that in such a short time the contagion that marches so slowly by itself and which is communicated with such difficulty, should overrun such a number of countries, after having been (as it is claimed), imported by a single fleet of Spanish ships. For it is well known that its existence was determined in Spain, France, Italy and Germany and all through Scythia at the same period of time. Without doubt the malady originated spontaneously, like the petechial fever, or it had always existed."

"A barber, my friend, has a very old manuscript, containing directions for the treatment of the affection. This has for its title: *'Medicine for the thick scabs, with pains in the joints.'* The barber remembered the remedy laid down in this work, and at the very commencement of the new malady thought he recognized the contagion by the name of the *thick* scabs. But physicians having examined this remedy found it too violent, inasmuch as it was composed of quicksilver and sulphur. He would have been happier had he not consulted the doctors; he would have grown wealthy by incalculable gains."

We see from this that the syphilis of the fifteenth century did not present precisely the same symptoms as the variety of to day. Formerly secondary and tertiary accidents supervened much more rapidly, besides being very violent in their manifestations. Besides the disease was exceedingly malignant often causing, death in a short time, which fact led many authors of that epoch to consider the symptoms due to a pestilence brought about by general causes.[40] Nicholas Massa wrote in fact, that: "The patient has pains in the head, arms, and especially the legs, which are always intensified at night. The buboes in the two groins are salutary when they suppurate. We observe a chafed and scaly condition of the palms of the hands and soles of the feet. Ulcers of a bad appearance are frequently noted on the penis; these ulcers are hard and callous and very slow in healing. In exploring the throat we often discover a relaxed condition of the uvula and the presence of sordid ulcers, which rarely suppurate. With all this eruptive process we note certain hard tumors that adhere to the skin and bone and bear the name of *gummata*. These tumors may ulcerate and produce osseous caries."[41]

We notice the same errors in all the descriptions given by the authors of the sixteenth century; they exhibit an imperfect knowledge of the symptomatology, of the genesis and primitive constitutional accidents. We see that as yet clinical medicine had no existence, and that our predecessors were ignorant of the art of co-ordinating the signs of a disease in a thoughtful manner. Nevertheless, their descriptive powers in writing on venereal diseases, as before noted, were excellent, and had the merit of exactitude and honest observation; as, Pierre Manardi observes: "The principal sign of the French disease consists in pustules coming out on the end of the penis in men and at the entrance of vulva or neck of womb among women. Most frequently these pustules ulcerate; I say frequently for the reason that I have seen patients in whom these ulcers were hard as warts, cloves or apple seeds."

Here we have the aspect of primary syphilis presented by a physician whose name will, with justice, remain attached to the disease as long as it has a history. The secondary symptoms of the malady have never been more dramatically pictured than by Fernel, who remarks: "They had horrible ulcers on them, which might be mistaken for glands, judging from size and color, from which issued a foul discharge of a villainous infecting kind, enough to give a heart-ache; they had long faces of a greenish-black complexion, so covered with sores that nothing more hideous could be imagined."[42]

Relative to the duration of secondary symptoms, under date of 1495, Marcello de Cumes wrote from the camp of Novarro that "the pustules on the face, like those of leprosy and variola, lasted a year or more when the patient was not treated."[43]

The physiognomy of the unfortunates whose faces were adorned with lumps and whose foreheads bore the sadly characteristic *corona veneris*, has been well described in the following verses by Jean Lemaire, of Belgium, a poet and historical writer of fifteenth century. The portrait is exact:

"But in the end, when the venom is ripe,

Sprout out big warts of a scarlet type,

Persistent, spreading over the face,

Leaving the brand of shame and disgrace,

An injury left after passion's rude storm,

Fair human nature thus to deform.

High forehead, neck, round chin and nose

Many a warty sore disclose;

And the venom, with deadly pain,

Runs through the system in every vein,

Causing innumerable ailments, no doubt,

From itch to the ever-tormenting gout," etc.

Meantime, the symptoms of syphilis were not long in losing some of their acute features. Already, in 1540, Antoine Lecocq noted this fact in France:[44] "Sometimes," says he, "the virus seems to expend its strength on the groins in tumefaction of the glands; and, if this bubo suppurates, it is well. This tumor we call bubo; others call it *poulain* (colt or filly) for mischief's sake, as those who are thus attacked separate their legs while walking, horse style." Fernel declared that the venereal disease at the end of the sixteenth century so little resembled that of his early days that he could scarcely believe it the same. He remarks: "This disease has lost much of its ferocity and acuteness."

On his part, Fracastor remarked, in 1546, that "For six years past the malady has changed considerably. We now notice pustules on but few patients, and they have but few pains, and these are generally slight; but more gummy tumors are observed. A thing that astonishes the world is the falling out of the hair of the head and baldness in other portions of the body. It sometimes happens that in the worst cases the teeth become loose and even fall out."[45]

These phenomena were evidently due to the action of mercurial ointment, which was much used in Italy from the time it was recommended by Hugo, of Boulogne, in the *malum mortuum*, or malignant leprosy of the Occident. In France guaiac was much used, or holy wood, which was then known as *sanctum lignum*, when only the Latin equivalent was in vogue. Besides, mention is made of mercurial stomatitis following inunctions with the so-called Neapolitain ointment in the Prologue of *Pantagruel*, by Rabelais.

This passage from Dr. Francis Rabelais[46] leads us to think that physicians were undecided about caring for syphilitic patients in the fifteenth century, almost all doctors, in fact, refusing to examine into the character of a disease of which they knew nothing; a disease whose infecting centers were the most degraded and ignoble public places; a malady not described in the works of Hippocrates nor Galen.

So, this *lues venerea*, as it is called by Fernel, made numerous victims in all countries. It spread in the towns and throughout the rural districts, and, at times, caused such ravages that, in the large cities, the authorities were obliged to use sanitary measures against the pox, as had been done at other times in the case of leprosy. Syphilitics were expelled from places and forbidden, under severe penalties, from having intercourse with healthy people. But it soon came to be known that contagion could only occur through sexual connection, and the patients then hid in hospitals, where they were specially treated by the methods laid down by the first syphilographers,—vapor baths, mercurial inunctions, frictions, etc. Unfortunately, no prophylactic measures were instituted against prostitutes, although they were recognized as having a monopoly in venereal disorders; for they did not believe at that time, like Jean de Lorme, who said: "The pox may be caught by touching an infected person; by breathing the same air; by stepping, barefooted, in the patient's sputa, and in many other manners."

Even the poets wrote sonnets, poems and ballads upon this *mal d'amour* (lovesickness). One could form an immense volume by collecting all the verses written and published on this subject during the sixteenth century. But no poem indited during that period presents so great an interest to medical science as the ballad of Jean Droyn, of Amiens, dedicated to the Prince, in which the author, stronger in the etiology of syphilis than the doctors of his time, advised young men who feared *grosse verole* (the pox) not to indulge in *liasons* with girls of the town without first being satisfied with their pathological innocence.

This ballad was published at Lyons in 1512, that is to say, seventeen years after the appearance of the disease in the army of Charles VIII., at an epoch when the majority of doctors considered the affection as an infectious malady due to the action of a pestilential miasm in the air. We shall reproduce but a few lines of this poetical-medical-historical document:

"Perfumed darlings, dandies, dudes,

Take warning in each case,

Beware all types of fleshy nudes

And don't fall in disgrace.

Sure, gentlemen and tradesmen gay

May throw away their money,

Give banquets and at gaming play,

As flies are drawn by honey.

I warn you all of love's sweet charms,

Place on them protocole,

For haunting oft strange women's arms

Brings sometimes *grosse verole*.

"Let love, with moderation wise,

Attend each amorous feast.

Let all be clean unto your eyes,

Fly all lewd girls at least.

Happier and nobler 'tis to gain

For virtue high renown

Than wound your honor with a stain,

With women of the town.

Keep out of danger from disease,

Good health will you console,

But if you strive the flesh to please

Beware of *grosse verole*."

In the final stanzas of this poem, which will not bear a more complete reproduction owing to a maudlin sentimentality existing in modern times, we find that the Prophet Job is not regarded as strictly virtuous, for we read:

"Prince, sachez que Job fut vertueux,

Mais si futil rongneux et grateleux,

Nous lui prions qu'il nous garde et console,

Pour corriger mondains luxurieux,

S'est engendree ceste grosse verole."

Notwithstanding the undoubted proof of the antiquity of venereal diseases, Astruc, as we all know, defends the American origin of the malady, and endeavors to support his views on the hypothesis emitted by Ulrich de Hutten in 1519, *i.e.*, at the siege of Naples, at the end of 1494, a Spanish army commanded by Gonsalva of Cordova came to the rescue of the besieged. Their soldiers communicated to the girls of the town and the courtesans of the neighborhood the *maladie Americaine* (American disease), which was contracted in turn, after the capture of Naples, by the army of King Charles, and afterwards spread throughout France. But history informs us that the King of France did not return to Paris with his troops from the Italian campaign until the month of March, 1496. Now it was on the 6th of March, in this same year, that Parliament issued a proclamation regulating the pox, in which the first section reads: "To-day, the 6th of March, whereas in the City of Paris a disease of a certain contagious character, known as *verole* (pox), prevails, the which has made much progress in the Realm the past two years, as well at Paris as in other places, and there is reason to fear, this being Springtime, that it may increase, it is deemed expedient to take cognizance of the same."

Other testimony is gathered from the narrative of the voyages of Christopher Columbus by his contemporary Petrus Martyr, of Anghierra, historian attached to the court of Ferdinand and Isabella. According to the notes given him by the great navigator on his return to Spain, authentic records kept from day to day,[47] the Spanish and Italian sailors of Columbus found "people who lived in the Age of Gold; with no ditches, no fences, no books, no laws. The men were entirely naked, the women only protected by a belly-band of light material; notwithstanding all this, their morals were pure." Besides, Petrus Martyr (*La Syphilis au XV. Siecle*) proves there was syphilis in Spain in 1487.

When Columbus returned to Europe a second time he left behind him, under orders of his brother, a hundred of his companions in arms, who were a collection of adventurers from all the nations of the earth. These men committed all sorts of excesses among the unfortunate Indians—steeping themselves in lust and every manner of crime, violating the women, and indulging in wholesale debauchery. Says Charles Renaut: "Looking at matters from this standpoint, I am ready to believe that the Spaniards carried the disease to the natives of Hispanola, and that the latter did not give the malady to the Spanish."

We shall not dwell further on the origin of syphilis, nor its connection with leprosy and other cutaneous maladies which were so prevalent in Europe throughout the Middle Ages. We may consider the disease as something new, and trace its period of invasion and development to the discovery of America, or assert that it arose from a semi extinct affection (leprosy), assuming a new type under the influence of a special epidemic constitution.

One thing is clearly proven, *i.e.*, that syphilis was preceded by contagious venereal affections, which lost the irregular and malignant forms of the fifteenth century. When then the civilized nations of earth create a true Public Health Service, syphilis will be vanquished, and will pass away to the ranks of other extinct maladies.

THE DEMONOMANIA OF THE MIDDLE AGES.

ORIGIN OF MAGIC AND SORCERY

From the day that Louis XIV. dissolved the Parliament of Rouen, which had condemned several persons in the Province of Vire to death for the crime of sorcery, but few sorcerers have been seen in France.

It was in 1682 that Urbain Grandier was tortured and burned alive for having launched a malediction against the Ursulines of Loudun.

A violent reaction occurred against the Inquisitors, theologians, and their accomplice butchers, thanks to the courageous intervention of eminent philosophers and savants, who were justly indignant at the crimes of the Roman Catholic priesthood. This reaction clearly demonstrated the fact that the innumerable victims of religious intolerance in the Middle Ages were not sorcerers, nor possessed of the devil, nor minions of Hell. Psychologists and moralists claimed that the victims of these delusions were insane, persons suffering from semi delusions, subjects of monomania. Science classed these unfortunates into several groups, among which may be enumerated persons afflicted with hallucinations, demonomaniacs, erotomaniacs, subjects of lycanthropy, etc., without counting vampires, choreomaniacs, lypemaniacs, and others whose attacks are recognized by medical science.

The encyclopedists and their disciples declared themselves satisfied, inasmuch as psychological experts had done away with the absurd traditions of the Middle Ages as well as antique superstitions. The death penalty for demonidolatry was removed, but the doors of the insane asylum opened for its followers.

Could any better arrangement have been made at the present day? Let us take the history of this famous epidemic of demonidolatry of other days and examine the documentary evidence offered against those accused of the crime of sorcery, passing the testimony through the crucible of modern science, pathology, physiology, together with all observable symptoms, holding in view meanwhile modern neurological discoveries; let us strive, in a word, to solve this great psychological question, which has greatly agitated the human understanding for four hundred years past.

We believe *what is, is the truth*, and in order to best judge the facts narrated, it is well to first arrange our knowledge as to the psychological condition of Occidental populations during the Middle Ages, a condition that was only the continuation of the ideas and traditions of antiquity, modified by the fanatical prejudices of a new religion and by a cruel and barbarous social Constitution.

If history authorizes us, in fact, to conclude that the occult sciences have existed from the earliest periods of antiquity, that the people who brought learning from the Orient to the Occident, have at all times admitted the existence of genii, angels, and demons, it is easy to explain the action that such mysterious traditions would have on the ignorant minds of the peasantry of the Middle Ages, bowed under the yoke of slavery to feudal Lords and the clerical despotism of the Romish Church.

Let us interrogate these historical texts with impartiality, and analyze these ancient theogonies, which are, so to speak, the *proces verbaux* of the philosophic development of the human mind, and we shall see whether we can admit that mental diseases may prevail *epidemically* for several generations, like the pestilential maladies of the fourth century, for example.

We know that it was in India, the cradle of human genius, that the doctrine of supernaturalism, of good and bad spirits exerting an occult influence on mankind, was born. Ancient history shows such a belief goes back to antique times. Zoroaster, inspired by *Ahura Mazda*, the Omniscient, wrote, in the Zend Avesta, the text and commentaries of the religious law dedicated to the Aryas of India and Persia. This law had for its object the destruction of the cult of *dews* or demons, who infested the earth under human forms, and also to repress the naturalistic instinct of the most ancient people of *Asia*, by initiating them in a faith for Celestial genii.

The disciples of Zoroaster were the *Magi*; that is to say, the learned men of the day, but they modified the doctrine of the Prophet, which the Guebres alone preserved in its purity, with the fundamental doctrine of the dualism of light and darkness, represented by *Ormazd* and *Ahriman*, the spirit of the blest and the spirit of the damned.

The Chaldeans, celebrated from times of antiquity for their knowledge, not only of astronomy, but all other sciences, adopted the doctrines of the Zend-Avesta, and their Magi transmitted the same to the Egyptians, Hebrews, Greeks, and Romans, and finally to the Gauls, whose adepts were the Druids.

The science or Magic of the Chaldeans was only magnetism, somnambulism, and spiritism.

Says M. F. Fabart: "The Magi, according to certain *bas reliefs* exhumed in Oriental countries, knew the virtue of magnetic passes. We see figures with hands extended, influencing by their gestures the subjects, who, seated before them, have closed eyes.

"The Pythonesses and Sybills did not have the power of foresight until they had passed through the crisis of an artificial somnambulism, and we find passages in antique authorities where this imposed sleep is discussed.[48]

In one of my preceding works I have spoken of several very curious passages in the *Pharsalia* of Lucan, where he speaks of the oracles of the female magician Erichto and the responses of the Pythonesses in the Temple of Delphi to the inquiries of Appius. Cassandra, priestess to Apollo in the tragedy of Agamemnon, by Seneca the tragedian, is a perfect type of the hypnotizable hysteric, and, if the poet does not describe the methods followed by the priests of the temple in order to magnetize their subjects, we find them noted by other Latin authors in terms so explicit as to leave no doubt as to their knowledge of magnetic passes (hypnotism).

Says Cœlius Aurelianus: "We make circular movements with the hands before the eyes of the patient. Under our gaze the subject follows the movements of our hands, the eyes blinking." It is while giving the treatment for catalepsy that the Roman physician, the contemporary of Galen, initiates us in magnetic practice. After giving a description of the neurosis, which he characterizes by prostration, immobility, rigidity of neck, loss of voice, stupor of the senses, widely opened eyelids, fixity of the eyes and ocular expression, the Latin author teaches us how to relieve the disease and partially waken the movement, senses, and intelligence of the patient; and he magnetizes, as is clearly indicated in the following lines: "*Atque ita, si ante oculos eorum quisquam digitos circum moveat, palpebrant ægrotantes, et suo obtutu manuum trajectionem sequuntur; vel si quicquam profecerint etiam toto obtutu converso attendunt; et inclamati, respicientes lacrymantur nihil dicentes, sed volentium respondere vultum æmulantes.*"[49]

The precepts of Zoroaster were differently modified among ancient people. Moses, who wished the glory of being the great prophet of Israel, wrote the law of Jehovah and abjured the Magi, by whom he had been initiated. The Hebrews meantime preserved the Mazadean religion in memory; they created magic. Ahriman became Astaroth, Beelzebub, Asmodeus and other demons, who had for interpreters the Pythonesses and Prophetesses (*mediums*). Ormazd was transferred into a legion of angels and archangels, who appeared to men to make prophecies. Presently the Jewish magicians invented the *Kabbala*, occult science, by which, in pronouncing certain words, they performed miracles and submitted supernatural powers to the caprices of the human will; they were above all necromancers.

The occult sciences of the ancients, necromancy and magic, had, as will be observed, more or less connection with the phenomena of magnetism of the present day. Meantime necromancy resembled modern spiritualism, toward which the researches of present day magnetizers tend. The necromancers invoked the souls of the dead to know the future and the secrets of the present. The Jews pursued this study with much ardor, notwithstanding the prohibition of Moses, who wished them not *to speak to wood*. We know that the Pythoness (*witch*) of Endor evoked the spirit of Samuel before Saul on the eve of battle and predicted the King's death. The grotto where this celebrated medium lived still exists, and she receives, it is said, the travelers who visit her from far and wide near Mount Tabor.

Magic was also known by the High Priests in Pharaoh's court. Like the Magi of Medea and Chaldea they invoked the spirits and supernatural powers by methods and ceremonies consisting principally of gestures and songs.

Hermes Trismegistus, whom the Alchemists regard as their master, spread the science of occult magic. Following him we see the mystical doctrines of the Orient flourish at Alexandria with the founders of neoplatonism. These taught that the *Goetie* was the supernatural art which is practiced by the aid of wicked spirits, that the *Magie* produced mysterious manifestations with the assistance of material demons and superior spirits; that the *Pharmacists* controlled spirits by means of philters and elixirs.

In Greece and in Italy the celestial genii were believed in, and they multiplied to infinity, peopling the Olympus of Polytheism. Priests profited by the superstitious idea of the people who invoked the aid of the witches and sibyls who derived their wisdom from the Magi of the Orient. Following the example, the historians, philosophers and poets were apparently led to the belief in all the Genii, in the power of spirits and their intimate relations with men through the medium of seers, in a condition of frenzy or somnambulism (trance).

We know that the poet Hesiodus in his theogony, that Plato, from the time of his initiation with the Hermetic doctrines, that Aristotle in his philosophical works, all admit the existence of immaterial beings interesting themselves in the affairs of humanity. The Pythagorians, on their side, affirmed their power of controlling demons by keeping themselves in constant meditation, abstinence and chastity.[50]

During all times of antiquity, there were corporations of priests, philosophers, theosophists, thaumaturgists and other sects, who exercised the trade of invoking spirits by conjuring them with charms, by enchantments and witchcraft, and changing by their aid the laws of nature, to command the elements and accomplish other extraordinary feats. In order to do these prodigies they had recourse to cabalistic formulæ, indicated in conjuring books, or by incantations, magical circles, or simply by magnetic power.

Simon of Samaria, Circe, Medea, Plotinus, Porphyrius, Jamblichus, and the famous Canidie, so justly cursed by Horace, belonged to this clan of magicians, gnostics, enchanters and mediums, who acquainted the people with the occult arts of the magi of Chaldea. It is only necessary to study history to be convinced of this fact.

Damis, the historian and pupil of Apollonius of Tyana, has left us the biography of his master, the most remarkable thaumaturgist of antiquity. It is in this work that he shows that while Apollonius was lecturing on philosophy at Ephesus, he stopped in the midst of his speech and cried out to the murderer who, at the same moment, assassinated Domitian at Rome, "Courage, Stephanus; kill the tyrant!" Apollonius had sojourned long in India, and all his disciples have attested the marvelous things he could do. He cured incurable diseases and made other miracles that astonished his contemporaries who were partisans, like himself, of the doctrines of Pythagoras.

Porphyrius published the fifty-four treatises of his master Plotinus, the illustrious neoplatonist, a work in which we find all the ideas of contemporaneous experimental psychology and a mystical philosophy supported on extasy, contemplation and hypnotism—ideas which were again enunciated one day by the enchanter Merlin, Albertus Magnus, Pic de la Mirandolle, Lulle, Cornelius Agrippa, Count Saint Germain, Joseph Balsamo, Robert Fludd, Richard Price and the *freres* of *Rose Croix*.

But, before these, there were others who believed they preserved the mysterious secrets of nature, the Illuminati, the seers and others not our immediate ancestors; the Druids in the dark forests of Gaul, along with the Druidesses. Both classes belonged to the Sacerdotal order, and only received the vestures of their sacred ministry after twenty years consecrated to the study of astrology, laws of nature, medicine and the Kabbala. Their theodicy taught the existence of one God alone and the immateriality of the spirit, called after death to be reincarnated an indetermined number of times up to the point when perfection was obtained; when a new, more divine and happy distinction was achieved. It admitted as a principal religious dogma the ascendant metempsychosis, as in the case of the first magi and the great Greek philosophers; also a multitude of genii and superior spirits intermediate between the Divinity and mankind.

The *Druids* were not only the priests, but dictators of Gaul; they were assisted in their functions by the *Eubages*, the soothsayers and sacrifices of their religion, by the *Bards*, the poets and heralds, and the *Brenns*, who participated in supreme power. Druidism was then an admixture of warlike ideas of the first inhabitants of Gaul, together with the doctrines imported by the Magii from Chaldea. So the Druids were the astronomers, physicians, surgeons, priests and lawgivers. The Druidesses, descendants of the Pythonesses and Sibyls of the Orient, spoke in oracles and predicted the future; their influence was considerable and often surpassed that of the Druid priests themselves, for they knew just as well how to use the Kabbala and magic; and besides, as virgins, consecrated depositaries of the secrets of God, they stood high in the eyes of the people. It is for this reason that the Druids and Druidesses were, under Roman domination, the defenders of national independence; but, forced to take refuge in dense forests far removed from the people, persecuted by the Romans, barbarians and Christians, they progressively became magicians, enchanters, prophets and charmers, condemned by the Councils and banished by civil authority.

It is at this epoch that evil spirits were noticed prowling around in the shadows of night and indulging in acts of obscene depravity. There were the *Gaurics*, beings the height of giants; the *Suleves*, beardless personages who were succubi, attacking travelers; and the *Dusiens* were incubi, demons who deflowered young girls during their maiden slumbers.

Saint Augustin accorded his belief to all these fables, which were retailed throughout the country, affirming that we have no right to question the existence of these demons or libertine spirits, which make impure attacks on persons while asleep. (*Hanc assidue immunditiam et tentare et efficere,*—Saint Augustin, in his "City of God.")

Decadence slowly ensued, so that in the seventh century Druidism disappeared, but the practice of magic, occult art, and the mysterious science of spirits were transmitted from generation to generation, but lessened in losing the philosophic character of ancient times. In a word, magic became sorcery, and its adepts were no longer recruited save in the infamous and ignorant classes of society. The adoration of nature and God, the immortality of the soul, the grand ceremonies held at the foot of gigantic oak trees, gave way to hideous demons, gross superstitions, witchcraft, and the most immoral abberations. Occultism still subjugated the masses, but the science had fallen into the hands of the profane and of charlatans.

THE THEOLOGIANS AND DEMONOLOGICAL JUDGES.

Magic, or the science of magic, then served as a basis, as we have said before, for mythology and legends and was noticeable in the dogmas of all religions, for, as Saint Augustin observes, "In order to penetrate the mystical senses of fictions and allegories, and the parables contained in sacred history, it is necessary to be versed in the study of occult science, of which numerals make part."[51]

But from the Greek dæmon, or the *Sapiens* of Plato, Christianity made a demon, a fallen angel, who wished to people his empire with the souls of the unbaptized; he is borrowed from the Jews with Beelzebub, Asmodeus, Satan, and their numerous colleagues. After Jesus, who was tempted by the Devil, and who delivered those possessed by devils, we see the apostles and saints visited in turn by the angels of God and also by spirits of evil, who fight battles among spiritual armies. These are only visions, apparitions of angels or demons who are vanquished before the anointed of the Lord.

Mankind wished to participate in the honors and emotions of communicating with supernatural beings; it is for this purpose that humanity addressed magicians and practitioners of Occultism. So we see in the first ages of Christianity the Bishops were uneasy in regard to magicians by reason of the popularity of the latter, notwithstanding the peasantry had submitted to the dogmas of the Church.

Paul Lacroix, the learned bibliophile, cites as the most ancient monument made mention of in this connection, an aggregation of shadowy women collected for a mysterious purpose, who devoted themselves to making magical incantations; this fragment is gathered from the Canons of a Council which, he thinks, was held before the time of Charlemagne. It treats of aerial flights that these sorcerers made, or thought they made, in company with Diana and Herodias, *i.e.*, "*Illiud etiam non est omitendum quod quædam sceleratæ mulieres, retro post Satanam conversæ, demonum illusionibus et phantasmatibus seductæ, credunt et profitentur se nocturnis horis, cum Diana, dea paganorum, vel cum Herodiate et innumera multitudine mulierum, equitare super quasdam bestias, et multarum terrarum spacia intempestæ noctis silentio pertransire ejusque jussionibus velut dominæ obedire, et certis noctibus ad ejus servitium evocari.*"[52]

Which, being freely translated, reads: "We must not forget that impious women devoted to Satan, were seduced by apparitions, demons and phantoms, and avowed that during the night they rode on fantastic beasts along with Diana, a Pagan goddess, or Herodias and an innumberable throng of women. They pretended to traverse immense space in the silence of the night, obeying the orders of the two demon-women as those of a sovereign, being called into their service on certain given occasions."

We can understand from this that if Christianity silenced Pagan oracles, it did not authorize magicians to put the spiritual world aside. The clergy accepted the evidence of the witnesses of grace, but refused that of the profane, who were only inspired by demons; they recognized in the latter the power of giving men illusions of the senses, of cohabiting with virgins under the form of *incubi* and with men under the form of *succubi*,—demons who could insinuate themselves through natural orifices into all the cavities of the body, and possess mortals.

Theologians have described all the pains endured by those possessed,— pangs in their thoracic and abdominal organs which, made by the demons, forced their victims to speak, sing, move, to be in a condition of anæsthesia or hyperæsthesia, following the imp's will; in other words, the possessed were subject to infernal action. To the worship of spirits the first Bishops of the Church substituted a foolish fear of demons.

From this exaggeration of the power of evil genii over man surged the silly terrors and superstitious fears of damnation, which were the starting-point of aberration among the first demonomaniacs. It was for these unfortunates that the clergy invented exorcisms and great annual ceremonies destined to deliver those possessed by demons, ceremonies at which the Bishops convened the people and the nobles to assist, in order to show the triumphs of the Church over Satan and his imps.

The theatrical arrangement of these assemblages certainly induced some apparent cures—making the faithful cry out "a miracle, truly;" but who does not know that all affections of the nervous system love to be treated at the hands of thaumaturgists? To invent demons to have the glory of defeating them and to deliver mankind from their influence,—such appears to have been the objective point of the primitive Christian Church. This was certainly a clever trick in theological magic, and, if the end did not seem to justify the means to critical philosophic eyes, we may admit, at least, that it was better to exorcise the possessed than to burn them alive at the stake, as was done some centuries later.

"This doctrine of demons was so intimately intermixed with the dogmas of this perfected religious system by the Fathers of the Church," says Sprengel, that "it is not astonishing authors attributed many phenomena of nature to the influence of demons." One of the most celebrated doctors of the Church, Origen, of Alexandria, in his *Apology for Christianity*, remarks: "There are demons that produce famines, sterility, corruption of the air, epidemics; they flutter surrounded by fogs in the lower regions of the atmosphere, and are drawn by the blood of their victims in the incense that the pagans offer them as their Divinity. Without the odor of sacrifice, these demons could not preserve their influence. They have the most exquisite senses, are capable of the greatest activity, and possess the most extended experience."

Saint Augustin had already written that demons were the agents of the diseases of Christians, and attacked even the new-born who came to receive baptism.

The Church taught that these demons acted through the intermediary of fallen creatures who were in revolt against God and his holy ministers. Such were the sorcerers and female mediums, who were met among ruins, in rocky cavern, and in other hidden and obscure places. For a morsel of bread or a handful of barley such creatures could be consulted; one could demand from them the secrets of the future, instruments for revenge, charms to secure love.

Among these sorcerers there were old panderers, who knew, from personal experience, all practices of debauchery, and who gave the name of *vigils* to the saturnalia indulged in among villagers on certain nights, gatherings composed of bawds and pimps, to which were invited numerous novices in libidinousness. These sorcerers and witches also knew the remedies that young girls must take when they wish to destroy the physiological results of their imprudences, and what old men need to restore their virility. They knew the medicinal qualities of plants, especially those that stupified. Perhaps a few of these sorcerers discovered, from magical incantations, the epoch of deliverance from Feudal morals, the abolition of servitude, equality and liberty. One thing is certain, however, *i.e.*, that the clergy saw nothing in them save enemies of the Church and religion, creatures who were dangerous to society and deserving only destruction, *per fas et nefas*, by exorcism, by fire— indeed, even by the accusations tortured out of insane persons.

Thus, Pope Gregory IX., in a letter addressed to several German Bishops in 1234, described the initiation of sorcerers as follows: "When the master sorcerers receive a novice, and this novice enters their assembly for the first time, he sees a toad of enormous size—as large, in fact, as a goose. Some kiss its mouth, others its rear. Then the novice meets a pale man, with very black eyes, and so thin as to appear only skin and bones; he kisses this creature, too, and feels a chill as cold as ice. After this kiss it is easy to forget the Catholic faith. The sorcerers then assemble at a banquet, during which a black cat descends from behind a statue that is usually placed in the center of the gathering. The novice kisses the rear anatomy of this cat, after which he salutes, in a similar manner, those who preside at the feast and others worthy of the honor. The apprentice in sorcery receives in return only the kiss of the master; after this the lights are extinguished and all manner of impure acts are committed among the assemblage."[53]

This was the belief, then, of those who a few years later composed the "*Tribunal of the Inquisition*" and accepted the banner of Loyola, and shortly afterwards again a member of the congregation of Saint Dominick and professor of theology, Barthelemi de Lepine, convinced of the existence of demons and Demonidolators, showed himself to be a furious adversary of the sorcerers in a famous dissertation, which was immediately adopted by his co-religionists. He affirmed that "the *possessed* go to the *sorcerers'* meetings in body or in spirit and have carnal intercourse with the devil; that they immolate children, transforming them into animals notably cats; that they have obscene visions, and it is best to exterminate them, for their number is growing legion."

Barthelemi de Lepine, in speaking thus, only followed the traditions of the Fathers of the Church; of Saint George, Saint Eparchius, Saint Bernard, Innocent VIII., and of Antonio Torquemada, who were the historians of the *incubi* of their times, and launched anathemas against the *possessed* of the Demon of luxury.

The Jesuit father Costadau wrote, in his treatise *De Signis, apropos* of incubism: "The thing is too singular to treat lightly. We would not believe it ourselves had we not been convinced by personal experience with the Demon's malice, and, on the other hand, find an infinity of writings of the first order from Popes, theologians, and philosophers, who have sustained and proved that there are men so unfortunate as to have shameful commerce and other things more execrable with such demons."

Another Jesuit, Martin Antoine del Rio, published six books (*Disquisitiones Magicæ*) in 1599, in which his credulity attained the limit of fanaticism, thus making the good priest one of the most redoubtable enemies of demonomania. Such were the doctrines on which reposed the theocratical pretensions of the theologians.

It is not astonishing that the last years of the Middle Ages, during the time religious struggles reached their highest period of exacerbation, owing to the quarrels between the Court of Rome and the Reformation, witnessed the multiplication in the number of demonomaniacs to such an extent that the whole world commenced to believe in the power of demons. "At this unfortunate time," remarks Esquirol, "the excommunicated, the sorcerers and the damned were seen everywhere; alarmed, the Church created tribunals, before which the devil was summoned to appear and the *possessed* were brought to judgment; scaffolds were erected, funeral pyres were lighted around stakes, and demonomaniacs, under the names of sorcerers and possessed, doubly the victims of prevailing errors, were burnt alive, after being tortured to make them renounce pretended compacts made with the Evil One. There was a jurisprudence against sorcery and magic as there were laws against theft and murder. The people, seeing the Church and Princes believing in the reality of these extravagances, were positively persuaded as to the existence of demons."

No authority raised itself to protect these miserable possessed people; justice, philosophy, and science remained subjected to theology, becoming more and more the accomplices of an autocratic and ever-intolerant Church.

Among the magistrates, historians and publicists, who were the most ardent supporters of the Inquisition, we may mention J. Bodin, of Angers, who published, in 1581, a work entitled *Demonomanie.* He shows that the victims of demonomania enjoy perfect integrity of the mental faculties and are in every sense responsible, before Courts of Ecclesiastical Justice and Parliaments, for their impure relations with supernatural beings, and he logically concludes that all Demonomaniacs should be committed to the stakes and burnt alive. "Meantime," says this amiable author, "we can deliver the possessed by exorcisms, and animals may be thus exorcised as well as men." To the support of his thesis he then brings an immense collection of ridiculous stories, which are not supported by evidence. He says: "Those possessed by a demon can spit rags, hair, wood and nails from their mouths."

He cites the case of a possessed woman who had her chin turned towards her back, tongue pushed out of the mouth, a throat which furnished sounds analogous to the crowing of a crow, the chatter of a magpie and the song of the cuckoo. Finally, he pretends that the devil may speak through the mouth of the possessed and use all the idioms, known and unknown; that he can deflower young girls and give them voluptuous sensations, etc.

This work of J. Bodin is, in reality, the argument of a public prosecutor, presented with passion and prejudice, having all the erroneous arguments of the Inquisitors, so that the latter were more than satisfied at convincing the secular magistrates and fixing their jurisdiction as to the crime of sorcery. On the other hand, the same year that Bodin gave publicity to his inhuman side of the question, the *Essays of Michel Montaigne* appeared in Paris, in which this celebrated writer appealed to philosophy. He demanded that human life should be protected from fantastic accusations, and made that famous response to a Prince who showed him some sorcerers condemned to death: "In faith, I would rather prescribe hellebore than hemlock faggots, as they appear to be more insane than culpable." Montaigne concluded one of his essays on this subject with the satirical remark: "It is placing a high valuation on human conjecture when we cook a man alive for an opinion."

Meantime, Bodin had reasoned against Montaigne. But the one remained the ignorant prosecutor of the Middle Ages, while the other was an immortal philosopher, whom Colbert certainly quoted before presenting to Louis XIV. the famous edict of 1682, which forbade in the future *"the cooking alive of sorcerers."*

Meantime, there was still a century to attain before one of the Prime Ministers of France put an end to all trials for sorcery, and during the intervening period there were other purveyors of the death penalty by the stake-burners of the Inquisition; among these were the celebrated Boguet, Criminal Judge of Bourgogne, and Pierre de l'Ancre, his colleague of Aquitanus, cited by Calmeil as the most fanatical judges of their day.

Boguet, in his *Discours des Sorciers*, wrote: "There were in France only three hundred thousand under King Charles IX., and they have since increased more than half as much again. The Germans prevent their growth by burning at the stake; the Swiss destroy whole villages at one time; in Lorraine the stranger may see thousands existing with but few executions. It is difficult to understand why France cannot purge itself of these creatures. These sorcerers walk around by thousands and multiply on earth like caterpillars in our gardens. I wish I could enforce punishment according to my ideas, for the earth would soon be purged of those possessed. For I fain would collect them all in one mass and burn them alive in a single bonfire."

Pierre de l'Ancre, Councillor to the Parliament of Bordeaux, published in 1613 his *Tableau de l'inconstance des mauvais anges et demons*, and in 1622 his *Incredulite et mecreance du sortilege pleinement convaincue*. In these two works the author treats all questions regarding sorcery, and declares that in his capacity of judge he believes it a mistake to spare the life of any individual accused of magic, as he considers sorcerers *as the enemies of morality and religion*, and accuses them of having found means of "ravishing women even while they laid in the embraces of their husbands, thus forcing and violating the sacred oaths of marriage, for the victims are made adulterous even in the presence of their husbands, who remain motionless and dishonored without power to prevent; the women mute, enshrouded in a forced silence, invoking in vain the help of the husband against the sorcerer's attack, and calling uselessly for aid; the husband charmed and unable to offer resistance, suffering his own dishonor with open eyes and helpless arms.

"The sorcerers dance around the bed in an indecent manner, like at a Bacchanalian feast, accoupling adulterously in a diabolical fashion, committing execrable sodomies, blaspheming scandalously, taking insidious carnal revenges, perpetrating all manner of unnatural acts, brutalizing and denaturalizing all physical functions, holding frogs, vipers, and lizards, and other deadly animal poisons in their hands, making stinking smells, caressing with lascivious amorousness, giving themselves over to horrible and shameful orgies."

Thus says the Prosecutor of the Council of Bordeaux, but he fails to support his statements by a single material fact, not even one individual case being proven. His trials show nothing but a few poor demented women, who responded always in the affirmative to the obscene and indecent questions of the judges and prosecutors *employed by the Most Holy Inquisition*.

A sad thing philosophy registers celebrated names during this Age. We mention only those of Rene Descartes, Blaise Pascal, Nicholas Malebranche, Thomas Hobbes, Francis Bacon, Leibnitz, and the immortal Newton. Unfortunately these great geniuses could not take part in the struggle between the clerical party and free thinkers. Honored as scholars, their Governments never asked their advice on questions claimed to be under the control of religious orders. The clergy had all the latitude they desired in writing the history of demonology, and also the evidence wrung from those accused of sorcery—vague responses drawn out by fear, by torture, by suggestion imposed in the obscurity of a penitential tabernacle. A witness of veracity, as we have before stated, never gave testimony as to the conduct of the sorcerers at the secret vigils. Their invocations on initiation, their famous inunctions used on the body, with magical ointments while in a condition of absolute nudity; their equestrian position on broom sticks; their flying tricks up the chimney and their bewitched reunions when horned devils rode on their shoulders, are legendary recitals which could only be accepted by ignorant fanatics and judges firm in the Faith. How a man with the seeming intelligence of Prosecutor Bodin, who was delegated by the State, who wrote six works on *The Republic* and *The Constitution*—works which have been compared in point of ability as ranking with Montesquieu's *Spirit of the Law*; how a publicist of talent could support such stories as we have mentioned in his work on sorcery is a matter of profound amazement. Yet, Bodin testifies as to his faith in the story of that peasant of Touraine "who found himself naked, wandering around the fields in the morning," and who gave as an explanation of his conduct that he had surprised his wife the night before as she was making preparations to go to a sorcerers' vigil, and that he had followed his better half, accompanied by the Devil, as far as Bordeaux, many leagues away. Bodin also believed the narration of that girl from Lyons "whom the lover perceived rubbing herself with magical ointment preparatory to attending a sorcerers' vigil; and the lover, using the same ointment, followed his girl and arrived at the vigil almost as soon as she."

As to that poor peasant who was found naked and alone in the field and forced to denounce his wife to the authorities, Bodin remarks impressively, "The woman confessed and was condemned to be burnt at the stake."

Pierre de l'Ancre was never able to prove his stories by sentinels, sergeants, guards, or policemen, as to the appearance of the demon he described in his *Traite sur les demons*; a spirit that showed itself as a large blood-hound or as a wild bull. It is true that in another part of his book he demonstrates the changeable character of his Devil, and gives the following description, which methinks is more worthy the pen of an insane man rather than that of a magistrate: "The Devil of the *sabbat* (vigil) is seated in a black chair, with a crown of black thorns, two horns at the side of the head and one in the forehead with which he gores the assemblage. The Devil has bristling hair, pale and troubled looking face, large round eyes widely opened, inflamed and hideous looking, a goatee, a crooked neck, the body of a man combined with that of a billy goat, hands like those of a human being, except that the nails are crooked and sharp pointed at the ends; the hands are curved backwards. The Devil has a tail like that of a jackass, with which, strange to say, he modestly covers his private parts. He has a frightful voice without melody; he preserves a strange and superb gravity, having the countenance of a person who is very melancholy and tired out from overwork."

This was the spirit of the lieutenants of justice called on by the Inquisitorial clergy to fix the penalty for the crime of sorcery. "Sorcery being a crime," say they with the spirit of conviction, "consented to between man and the Devil; the man bowing to adore Satan, and receiving in exchange a part of his infernal power."

According to this compact, "The demon unites carnally with the sorcerer and female medium likewise; these unite themselves with Satan, denying God, Christ and the Virgin, and profaning all objects of sanctity by their profane presence.

"They become zealots for evil and render eternal homage to the Prince of Darkness.

"They are baptized by the Devil and dedicate to his service all children born to them by nature.

"They commit incests, poison people, and bewitch and work cattle to death.

"They eat the carrion from the rotting bodies of hanged criminals.

"They enter into a Cabalistic circle laid out by the accursed one, and matriculate in a secret order which is engaged in all manner of outrages against society; they accept secret marks that affirm their complete vassalage to Satan.

"Finally, they repudiate all authority other than that of the master in the Cabala (Kabbala), and, abomination above all, *they incite the people to revolt.*"

Meantime, while the Judges and Inquisitors pursued all intelligent people with the most wicked determination, Leloyer published his monograph on specters,[54] whose doctrines are closely connected with modern Spiritualistic theories.

This celebrated Councillor wrote that the soul, the spiritual essence which animates the organism, may be distracted and separated from the body for an instant, as we see in cases of ecstacy.

Now, we know that this nervous phenomenon, which may be *natural,* when connected with catalepsy, hysteria and somnambulism, or *provoked* when it is produced experimentally on subjects in a hypnotic condition, almost always coincides with an acute moral impression and a suspension of one or more of the senses. It is during the duration of this phenomenon that the soul, according to Leloyer, performs far-off journeys,—not orthodox, however, for we are told that during the period of such ecstacies, following cataleptic immobility, seven of these ecstatics were burned alive at Nantes in 1549.

In another chapter, he adds that souls may, after death, impress themselves on our senses by taking fantastic forms. He supports this opinion by the incident relative to a daughter of the famous Juriscouncillor of the sixteenth century, Charles Dumoulin, who appeared to her husband and told him the names of assassins; and of the specter who informed the Justice of the crime committed by the woman Sornin on her husband, that the soul of Commodus appeared so often to Caracalla.

The author of the *Spectres* attributes to supernatural beings the frights experienced by certain persons who live in haunted houses. Every night they are awakened by the sound of noises,—blows resound on the floor and raps come on the partitions; every few minutes there are peals of ghostly laughter, whistling, clapping of hands to attract attention; these nervous persons see spirits and are startled at sudden apparitions of the dead; specters seize them by the feet, nose, ears, and even go so far as sit on their chests. Such houses are said to be the rendezvous of demons.

The persons spoken of by Leloyer *are to-day known as mediums producing physical effects*, and the phenomena observed centuries since are evidently the same as those investigated by William Crookes, with the collaboration of Kate Fox and Home.[55]

"In the ecstacy of sorcerers," resumes Leloyer, "the soul is present, but is so preoccupied by the impressions that it receives from the Devil, that it cannot act on the body it animates. On awaking, such ecstatics may remember things they have seen, events in which they have assisted, as in the case when the soul temporarily abandons its earthly tenement."

Meanwhile, it is but fair to observe that the author makes certain reservations; he admits that ecstacy and hallucination may be provoked by a pathological condition of the nervous system, and are not always the result of the work of demons. He also comments on a certain number of vampires remaining in a lethargic sleep, from a nervous condition, after returning from a sorcerer's vigil, a fact which, according to Calmeil, was of a nature to throw the theories of the Councillors of the Inquisition into disfavor.

The theory of the author of *Spectres* resembles considerably, as will at once be noticed, that of the first Magii and the modern doctrine of Spiritualism. Leloyer, besides, has gathered a number of facts to support his affirmations; among others, he cites the observation given him by Philip de Melanchton, the learned Hellenist and author of the famous confession of Augsburg. This was a spiritual manifestation experienced by the widow of Melanchton's uncle: One day, while weeping and thinking of the dear lost one, two spirits appeared to her suddenly,—"one habited in the stately, dignified form of her husband, the other specter in the garb of a gray friar. The one representing her husband approached her and said a few consoling words, touched her hand and disappeared with his monkish companion."

Melanchton, although one of the chiefs of the Reformation, was still imbued with the ideas of the Romish Church; after some hesitation he concluded that the specters seen by his aunt were demons. The same phenomena have been observed by modern *mediums*; William Crookes, the celebrated London scientist, relates facts to which he has been witness which are even more extraordinary than the one we have just narrated.

Jerome Cardan, of Paris, the celebrated mathematician, renowned for his discovery of the formula for resolving cubic equations, solemnly affirmed that he had a protecting spirit, and never doubted the reality of this apparition. Cardan also tells how his father one evening received a visit from seven specters, who did not fear to enter into an argument with the learned old man.

Imagination, exalted by chimerical fear of demons, sees the work of these evil-doing spirits on every hand, in gambling, in sickness, in accidents, in infirmity, in all the ordinary accidents of life. The sorcerers are accused of attacking man's virility by witchcraft. The victims say that some one has knotted their private organs (*noue l'aiguilette*). This pretended catastrophe in magic, the origin of which dates back to times of antiquity, may be classed among abnormal physiological effects under the influence of a moral cause, fear, timidity, and certainly the suggestion of a feeble mind.

Such are the sorcerers that Bodin accuses, perhaps not without reason always, since we see that impotency in some young melancholic subjects who appear easily impressed with fantastic notions.

"Sorcerers," says Bodin, "have the power to remove but a single organ from the body, that is, the virile organ; this thing they often do in Germany, often hiding a man's privates in his belly, and in this connection Spranger tells of a man at Spire who thought he had lost his privates and visited all the physicians and surgeons in the neighborhood, who could find nothing where the virile organs had once been, neither wound nor scar; but the victim having made peace with the sorcerer, to his great joy soon had his treasure restored."

There was no need of this kind of witchcraft, *pour nouer l'aiguilette*, in a timid boy, already subjugated by fear of the devil. Certainly, if the sorcerers had ideas of that force which is known to-day as *suggestion*, they could very easily destroy the virile power of the subject by governing his will and thoughts, his physical and moral personality. When we can confiscate the physical anatomy of a man he is reduced to all manner of impotencies. Who will affirm that suggestion is not one of the mysteries of sorcery?

DEMONOLOGICAL PHYSICIANS.

After the theosophists, theurgists, and the priests, we will now interrogate the writings of the physicians of antiquity and of the Middle Ages, as to this question of spirits and their connection with the affairs of mankind.

We see that Galen is often drawn away by the beliefs of his time, to the most ridiculous prejudices and fancies, and that he is the defender of magical conjurations. He claimed that Æsculapius appeared to him one day in a dream and advised bleeding in the treatment of pleurisy by which he was attacked.

After Galen, Soranus of Ephesus used magical chants for curing certain affections. Scribonius Largus, a contemporary of the Emperor Claudius, indicated the manner of gathering plants, so that they might possess the strongest healing properties (the left hand must be raised to the Moon). Plants thus gathered cured even serpent bites. Archigenes suspended amulets on the necks of his patients. And although Pliny often declared that he wished "to examine everything in nature and not to speculate on occult causes" he reproduces in his works all the superstitious practices employed in medicine.

In the sixth century, Ætius, physician to the Court of Constantinople, acquired great surgical renown by the preparation of applications of pomades, ointments, and other topical remedies, in which superstition played a leading *role*.[56] Thus, in making a certain salve it was necessary to repeat several times in a low voice, "May the God of Abraham, Isaac, and Jacob accord efficacy to this medicine." If one had a foreign body in the throat it was necessary to touch the neck of the patient and say, "As Jesus Christ raised Lazarus, and Jonah came out of a whale, come out thou bone"; or, better still, "The Martyr Blase and the Servant of Christ commands thee to come out of the throat or descend to the stomach."[57]

After Ætius, we see Alexander of Tralles indulge in the same follies. In the colic he bids us use a stone on which is represented Hercules seated on a lion, a ring of iron on which was inscribed a Greek sentence, and, on the other, the diagram of the Gnostics (a figure composed of two equilateral triangles); and he adds that sacred things must not be profaned.

Against the gout, the same Alexander of Tralles recommended a verse from Homer, or, better still, to engrave on a leaf of gold the words *mei, dreu, mor, phor, teus, za, zown*. He conjured, by the words *Iao, Sabaoth, Adonai, Eloi*, a plant he employed in the same disease. In quotidian fever he advised an amulet made of an olive leaf on which was written in ink, *Ka Poi. A*.[58]

In the thirteenth century, Hugo de Lucques said a *Pater noster* and other prayers to the Trinity to cure fractures of the limbs. But in the following century astrology replaced the magic of religious superstition. Arnauld de Villeneuve attributed to each hour of the day a particular virtue which influenced, according to the influence of the horoscope, the different parts of the body. According to Arnauld, we can use bleeding only on certain days when such and such a constellation is in place, and no other time; but the position of the moon more particularly needed attention. The most favorable time for phlebotomy was when Luna was found in the sign of Cancer; but the conjunction of the latter with Saturn is injurious to the effects of medicines, and especially of purgatives.[59]

His contemporary, Bernard de Gordon (of Montpellier), gives as a sure method of hastening difficult accouchments the reading of passages from the Psalms of David. He explains the humors of certain hours of the day in the following manner: the blood in the morning moves towards the sun, with which it is in harmony; but it falls towards evening, because the greatest amount of sanguification occurs during sleep. In the third hour of the day the bile runs downwards, to the end that it may not make the blood acid;[60] the black bile moves at the ninth hour and the mucus towards evening.

The efficacy of precious stones for bewitching, and many other superstitious ideas, were likewise noted by medical authors, notably Italian writers, as, for instance, Michel Savonarola, Professor at Ferrara, one of the most celebrated physicians of his age. In Germany, Agrippa of Nettesheim, philosopher, alchemist and physician, had a predilection for magic and the occult sciences, if we are to judge from his works published in 1530 and 1531, *i.e.*, *De incertitudianæ et vanitate scientiarum*, *De occulta philosophia*, in which he mentions action induced at a distance and forsees the discovery of magnetism.

Like him, his contemporaries, Raymond Lulle, in Spain, and J. Reuchlin, published books on the Cabala (*Kabbala*), and, in Italy, Porta founded, at Naples, the *Academy of Secrets*, for the development of occult sciences, which are explained in his treatise *De Magia Naturali*.

At almost the same epoch, Paracelsus, Professor at Basle, claimed that he possessed the universal panacea; that he had found the secret of prolonging life, by magic and astrology, for he diagnosed diseases through the influence of the stars. After him, Van Helmont defended animal magnetism, and gave himself up to the study of occult science, in company with his student, Rodolphe Goclenius.

In the sixteenth century, Fernel, who, inasmuch as he was a mathematician and an astronomer, published his *Cosmotheria*, where he indicated the means of measuring a meridian degree with exactitude; his remarkable works on physiology (*De naturali parte medicinæ*, 1542), on pathology and therapeutics, which gave him the nickname of the French Galen. Fernel fully admitted the action of evil spirits on the body of man; he believed that adorers of the Demons could, by the aid of imprecations, enchantments, invocations and talismans, draw fallen angels into the bodies of their enemies, and that these Demons could then cause serious sickness. He compared the *possessed* to maniacs, but that the former had the gift of reading the past and divining the most secret matters. He affirmed that he had been witness of a case of delirium caused by the presence of the Devil in a patient, that which was denied by several doctors at the epoch.[61] He also believed in lycanthropy....

In the same century, another of our medical glories, Ambroise Pare, the Father of French surgery, also adopted the theory of the Inquisitors regarding sorcery in his works,[62] in which may be found his remarkable anatomical and surgical discoveries. We read the following quaintly conceived passage: "Demons can suddenly change themselves into any form they wish; one often sees them transformed into serpents, frogs, bats, crows, goats, mules, dogs, cats, wolves, and bulls; they can be transmuted into men as well as into angels of light; they howl in the night and make infernal noises as though dragging chains, *they move chairs and tables*, rock cradles, turn the leaves of books, count money, throw down buckets, etc., etc. They are known by many names, such as cacodemons, incubi, succubi, coquemares, witches, hobgoblins, goblins, bad angels, Satan, Lucifer, etc.

"The actions of Satan are supernatural and incomprehensible, passing human understanding, and we can no more understand them than we can comprehend why the loadstone attracts the needle. Those who are possessed by demons can speak with the tongue drawn out of their mouth, through the belly and by other natural parts; they speak unknown languages, cause earthquakes, make thunder, clear up the weather, drag up trees by the roots, move a mountain from one place to another, raise castles in the air and put them back in their places without injury, and can fascinate and dazzle the human eye.

"*Incubi* are demons in the disguise of men, who copulate with female sorcerers; *succubi* are demons disguised as women, who practice vile habits not only on sleeping, but wakeful men."

"Ambroise Pare," says Calmeil, "believed that demons *hoarded up all kinds of foreign bodies in their victims' persons*, such as old netting, bones, horse-shoes, nails, horsehair, pieces of wood, serpents, and other curious odds and ends, and cites the wellknown case of Ulrich Neussersser."

The celebrated surgeon concludes from this that "it was the Devil who made the iron blades and other articles found in the stomach and intestines of the unfortunate Ulrich."

What would Pare have thought had he seen the strange objects so commonly found by modern surgeons in ovarian cysts? How many demons would it take to produce the numerous objects noticed at the present day?

Happily these demonological physicians accepted purely and simply the suggestion that demons could act on men, and abandoned the victims to the tender mercy of the theologians and their tools the lawyers. Yet, even in this time of atrocities there were a few courageous physicians who struggled for humanity as against ecclesiastical despotism. Let us quote, according to Calmeil, one Francoise Ponzinibus, who destroyed one by one all the arguments that served to support the criminal code against demons. It was this brave doctor who dared to write that demonidolatry constituted a true disease; that all the sensations leading the ignorant to believe in *spirits* who adored the Devil were due to a depraved moral and physical condition; that it was false that certain persons could isolate their souls from their bodies at night and thus leave their homes for far off places inhabited by demons; that the accouplement of sorcerers and all the crimes attributed to them could not be logically supposed but must be legally proven; that it was cruel and atrocious to burn demented people at the stake for witchcraft.

Let us also quote from Andre Alciat, another courageous physician, who dared accuse an Inquisitor of murdering a multitude of insane people on the plea of witchcraft. He considered the vigil (*sabbat*) of sorcerers as an absurd fiction, and saw in so-called *possessed* only so many poor demented women given over to fanatical delusions and wild dreams.

Paul Zacchias, the author of "Medico-Legal Questions" (*Questiones Medico-legales*), a work in which he shows himself to be as wise an alienist as Doctor of Laws. The avowed and open enemy of supernaturalism, he boldly denounced the cruelties committed against the demented.

Let us finally inscribe on the roll of honor, with our respects, the name of Jean Wier,[63] or rather of Joannes Wierus, physician to the Duke of Cleves, who studied in Paris, where he received the degree of doctor, and was afterwards the disciple of Cornelius Agrippa, a partisan of demonology. Like the latter, Jean Weir believed in astrology, alchemy, the cabala, sorcerers and female mediums; likewise in demons who possessed control of human beings through magic power. But in his works that he published in 1560 he proclaims the innocence of those unfortunates punished for witchcraft, and declares them to have been insane and melancholic; likewise asserting that they could have been cured by proper treatment. He declares that he is fully persuaded that sorcerers, witches, and lycanthropic patients who were burned at the stake were crazy people whose reason had been overthrown; and that the faults imputed to these unfortunates were dangerous to none but themselves; that the possessed were dupes to false sensations that had been experienced during the time of their ecstatic transports or in their sleep.

Weir[64] insisted that the homicidal monomania attributed to the inhabitants of Vaud should not be credited, and was not except by fools and fanatics; while the so-called vampires, whose blood was shed on the banks of Lake Leman, the borders of the Rhine, and on the mountains of Savoy, had never been guilty of crimes, nor murders especially, and cites cases of condemnation where the *insanity* or *imbecility* of the victims was incontestible. He declares, in general, that all sorcerers are irresponsible, that they are insane, and that the devils possessing them can be combatted without exorcism. "Above all," says he to the judges and executioners, "do not kill, do not torture. Have you fear that these poor frightened women have not suffered enough already? Think you they can have more misery than that they already suffer? Ah! my friends, even though they merited punishment, rest assured of one thing, *that their disease is enough.*" Beautiful words, worthy of a grand philosopher. Born in the sixteenth century, he believed in magic and sorcery; but as a physician he pleaded for the saving of human life, and as a man he frowned down the crimes committed on the scaffold. "The duty of the monk," says he, "is to study how to cure the soul rather than to destroy it." Alas! he preached his doctrine in the barren desert of ecclesiastical fanaticism.

Although, less well known than those names just mentioned, we must not forget to note that group of talented men who contributed with Ponzinibus, Alciat, Zacchias and Jean Wier in the restoration to medicine of the study of facts, thus freeing the healing art of many speculative ideas derived from the Middle Ages; we allude to such men as Baillou, Francois de la Boe (*Sylvius*), Felix Plater, Sennert, Willis, Bonet, and many other gallant souls who assisted in freeing medicine from the religious autocracy that overshadowed it,—men who were the *avant couriers* of modern positivism.

Many of those who had preceded these writers had been learned men and remarkable physicians, to whom anatomy, clinical medicine and surgery owed important discoveries, but the majority of these were not brave enough to defend their intelligence against religious superstitions. In some instances, indeed, they were even the criminal accessories of the theologians and inquisitors. In acting in adhesion to Demonological ideas, their very silence on grand psychological questions evidences their weakness,—we are sorry to say this,—and lowers them from the high position of humanitarians; the masses of the people of the Middle Ages owed the majority of their medical savants nothing on the score of liberty of conscience.

THE BEWITCHED, POSSESSED, SORCERERS AND DEMONOMANIACS.

In order to fully comprehend the Demonomania of the Middle Ages, it is necessary to previously analyze the different elements composing the medical constitution of the epoch, and, investigate under what morbid influences such strange *neuroses* were produced.

These influences, we shall find from thence, in the state of intellectual and moral depression provoked by the successive pestilential epidemics, which, from the sixth century decimated the population of Western Europe; in the disposition of the human mind towards supernaturalism, which had invaded all classes of society; in the terrors excited by the tortures of an ever flaming and eternal hell; in the fright, caused by the cruel and atrocious decisions of brutal Inquisitors, and their fanatical tools, the officers of the law. We find too, that a frightful condition of misery had weakened the inhabitants of city and country, morally and physically, inducing a multitude of women to openly enter into prostitution for protection and nutrition, owing to the iniquity of a despotic regime; then too, there were added bad conditions of hygiene and moral decadence, so that intelligence was sapped and undermined, together with a breaking down of the vitality of the organism.

In the recital of the miseries of the Middle Age, made by a master hand, by an illustrious historian, who bases his assertions on antique chronicles whose veracity cannot be questioned, we read the following: "Society was impressed with a profound sentiment of sadness, it was as though a pall of grief covered the generation; the whole world given over to plagues; the invasion by barbarians; horrible diseases; terrible famines decimating the masses by starvation; violent wind storms; greyish skies with foggy days; the darkness of night casting its shroud everywhere; a cry of lamentation ascends to Heaven through all this gruesome period. That sombre witness, our contemporary Glaber, fully indicates the position of society devoured by war, famine and the plague. It was thought that the order of seasons and the laws of the elements, that up to that period governed the world, had fallen back into the original chaos. It was thought that the end of the human race had arrived."[65]

When the epidemic of Demonomania attacked the earth, at the end of the fifteenth century, more than ten generations had undergone the depressive action of the superstitions and false ideas spread broadcast by religion. Heredity had prepared the earth, the human mind being in an absolute condition of receptivity for all pathological actions. The education of children was confined to teaching them foolish doctrines, diabolical legends, mysterious practices that weakened their judgments. With the progression, from childhood to majority, a vague sentiment of uneasiness was experienced with a constant preoccupation on the subject of conscience and sin. In full adult age, as we have observed, came religious monomania, with acute sexual excitement, and persistent erotic ideas.

Arriving at this phase of the situation, some became theomaniacs, others demonomaniacs, saying they were possessed by sorcery, under the influence of genesic and other senses, with psychal hallucinations, and in some cases, psycho-sensorial illusions. These fictitious perception were produced either through the influence of the mind, assailed by supernatural conceptions, or by morbid impressions transmitted most often by the great sympathetic, or, finally, by an unknown action arising from the exterior.

Under the influence of these hallucinations, which manifested themselves in a state of somnambulism, or during physiological sleep, the recollection persisting to the after awakening, the Demonomaniac responded to those asking questions, that he had heard the confused noises made by the sorcerers at their *vigil*, had heard also the conversation of the devils, and had seen scenes of the wildest prostitution enacted by the demons; that fantastic animals were perceived; that strange odors of a diabolical nature, the savor of rotten meat, and corrupt human flesh, tainted blood of new born babes, and other noisome things had been smelled; that these effluvias were horrible, repulsive, nauseating, combined with the stink of sorcerers and the sulphurous vapors of magical perfumes; that he felt himself touched by supernatural beings who had the lightness of smoke or mist, and wafted away in the air. The hallucinations of the genital senses had led him to believe he had carnal connection, always of a painful nature, with succubi. When the victim to these delusions was a woman, she had the impression of having been brutally violated or deflowered, and some women declared they oftentimes experienced the voluptuous sensations of an amorous coition.

These hallucinations developed one after the other; those belonging to the anesthetized class, coming first, those belonging to the genesic class, coming last. The complexity of their symptoms produced what we call *dedoublement*, or a dual personality. Those *possessed*, claimed to be in the power of a demon, who entered their body by one of the natural passages, sporting with their person, placing itself in apposition with any place in their organism, proposing all sorts of erotic acts, natural and unnatural, whispering shameless propositions in their ears, blasphemy against God, forcing them to sign a contract with the Devil in their own blood.

The nervous state in which such weak minded creatures were found, victims to nocturnal hallucinations, insensibly induced a species of permanent somnambulism, during which they acquired a particularly morbid personality. They affirmed themselves to be sorcerers possessed by demons. When this personality disappeared, and the patient returned to a normal condition, a simple suggestion was all sufficient to cause the reappearance of the hallucination. This explains why so many individuals accused of sorcery, denied at first what they afterwards affirmed. When the Judge demanded with an air of authority, what they had done at the witch meeting, (*vigil*), they entered into a most precise recital of minute details, and all the circumstances surrounding the nocturnal reunions of demons and their victims; and, by reason of this crazy avowal, or so called confession were burned at the stake for participation in diabolical practices.

In the *Chronicles of Enguarrand, of Monstrelet*, a truthful and trustworthy historian of the incidents of his time, we find a description of the famous *epidemics* of sorcery in Artois, which caused such a multitude of victims to be burnt at the stake, by order of the Inquisition. The facts recounted by this celebrated writer support the interpretations we have given to these phenomena. He expresses himself as follows:

"In 1459, in the village of Arras, in the country of Artois, came a terrible and pitiable case of what we named *Vaudoisie*. I know not why." "Those possessed, who were men and women, said that they were carried off every night by the Devil, from places where they resided, and suddenly found themselves in other places, in woods or deserts, when they met a great number of other men and women, who consorted with a large Devil in the disguise of a man, who never showed his face. And this Demon read, and prescribed laws and commandments for them, which they were obliged to obey; then made his assembled guests kiss his buttocks; after which, he presented each adept a little money, and feasted them on wines and rich foods, after which the lights were suddenly extinguished, and strange men and women knew each other carnally in the darkness, after which they were suddenly wafted through space, back to their own habitations, and awakened as if from a dream.

"This hallucination was experienced by several notable persons of the city of Arras, and other places, men and women, *who were so terribly tormented, that they confessed*, and in confessing, acknowledged that they had seen at these witch reunions many prominent persons, among others, prelates, nobles, Governors of towns and villages, *so that when the judges examined them, they put the names of the accused in the mouths of those who testified*, and they persisted in such statements although forced by pains and tortures to say that they had seen otherwise, and the innocent parties named were likewise put in prison, and tortured so much, that confessions were forced from them; and *these too, were burned at the stake most inhumanely*.

"Some of those accused who were rich and powerful escaped death by paying out money; others were reduced into making confessions on the promise that in *case they confessed their lives and property would be spared*. Some there were indeed who suffered torments with marvelous patience, not wishing to confess on account of creating prejudice against themselves; many of these gave the Judges large bribes in money to relieve them from punishment. Others fled from the country on the first accusation, and afterwards proved their perfect innocence."[66]

Calmeil considers this narrative of so-called sorcery as a delirium, prevailing epidemically in Artois, where "many insane persons were executed," although he is forced to add: "these facts lead us to foresee what misfortunes pursued the false disciples of Satan in former times."

These neuroses of the inhabitants of Artois had already been observed, almost half a century previous, among a class of sectarians by the name of the *Poor of Lyons*. These people were designated in the Romanesque tongue as *faicturiers*, the word *faicturerie* meaning sorcerer, or one who believes in magic. Demonomania then evidently dated back to the very commencement of the Middle Ages.

The judgment of the tribunals of Arras, which condemned the sorcerers of Artois to be burned alive at the stake, is a curious document in old French, which merits a short notice at least, for it is supported on the following considerations, which were accepted as veracious, although merely the delirious conceptions of ignorant peasants:

"When one wished to go to the witch reunion (*vigil*), it was only necessary to take some magical ointment, rubbed on a yard stick, and also a small portion rubbed on the hands. This yard stick or broomstick placed between the legs, permitted one to fly where he willed over mountain and dale, over sea and river, and carried one to the Devil's place of meeting, where were to be found tables loaded down with fine eatables and drinkables. There was also the Devil himself, in the form of a monkey, a dog or a man, as the case might be, and to him one pledged obedience and rendered homage; in fact one adored the Devil and presented unto him his soul. Then the possessed kissed the Devil's rear—kissing it goat fashion in a butting attitude. After having eaten and taken drink, all the assemblage assumed carnal forms; even the Devil took the disguise of man or sometimes woman. Then the multitude committed the crime of sodomy and other horrible and unnatural acts—sins against God that were so wholly contrary to nature that the aforesaid Inquisitor says he does not even dare to name, they are too terrible and wicked ever to mention to innocent ears, crimes as brutal as they were cruel."[67]

Among these sorcerers there was a poet, a painter and an old Abbot, who passed for an amateur in the mysteries of Isis. Perhaps the Inquisition pursued such individuals as sorcerers and heretics, knowing them to be given over to debauchery. Similar things occurred as before said very early in the Middle Ages.([68])

As also before mentioned, there were demons who cohabited with women at night, and sometimes with men, called *incubi* and *succubi*, following as they were active, (*incubare*, to lie upon), or passive, (*sub cubare*, to lie under).

Calmeil has written, that virgins dedicated to chastity by holy laws were frequently visited by these demons, disguised in the image of Christ, or of an angel, or seraphim. Sometimes the Devil took the form of the Holy Virgin, and attempted to seduce young monks from paths of piety. "Having impressed the victims with the power of beauty," says the sage alienist,([69]) "the wicked demon then got into the bed of the young girl, or young man, as the case might be, and sought to seduce them through shameful practices. The Gods, so say the ancients, often sought the society of the daughters of

Princes; these pretended Gods were nothing but demons. A Devil possessed Rhea, under the form of Mars, and this succubus passed for Venus the day Anchises thought he cohabited with the Godess of beauty.

"The demon incubi accosted by preference fallen women, under the form of a black man, or goat. From times immemorial, damned spirits have attacked certain females, under the form of lascivious brutes. Hairy satyrs or shags, fauns and sylvains were only disguised incubi.

The connections between the *possessed* and *incubi* were often accompanied by a painful sensation of compression in the epigastric region, with impossibility of making the least movement, the victim could not speak or breathe. She had all the phenomena noticeable in an attack of nightmare. Meantime, some had different sensations. A nun of Saint Ursula, named Armella, said that she seemed "always in company with demons who tempted her to surrender her honor. During five months, while this combat lasted, it was impossible to sleep at night, by reason of the specters, who assumed varied and monstrous shapes."[70] This virtuous nun preserved her chastity notwithstanding the frightful ordeal.

Angele de Foligno accused the incubi, says Martin del Rio, of beating her without pity, of putting fire in her generative organs, and inspiring her with infernal lubricity. There was no portion of her body that was not bruised by the attack of these demons, and the lady was not able to rise from her bed.

Another nun, named Gertrude, cited by Jean Wier, avowed that from the age of fourteen years, she had slept with Satan in person, and that the Devil had made love to her, and often wrote her letters full of the most tender and passionate expressions. A letter was found in this poor nun's cell, on the 25th of March, 1565. This amorous epistle was full of the details of the Demon's nocturnal debaucheries.

Bodin, in his "Demonomania" gives the observation of Jeanne Hervillier, who was burned alive, by sentence of the Parliament of Paris. She confessed to her Judges, that she had been presented to the Devil, by her grandmother, at the age of twelve years. "A Devil in the form of a large black man, who dressed in a black suit and rode a black horse. This Devil had carnal intercourse with her, the same as men have with women, only without seed. This sin had been continued every ten, or fifteen days, even after she married and slept with her husband."

This same author reports many instances of the same kind. Among others, that of Madelaine de la Croix, Abbess of a nunnery in Spain, who went to Pope Paul III., confessing, that from the age of twelve years, she had relations with a demon, *in the form of a Moor*, and, that for more than thirty years this commerce had been continued. Bodin firmly believes, that this nun had been presented to Satan, *"from the belly of her mother,"* and affirms that "such copulations are neither illusions, nor diseases." In his work, he also gives extracts of the interrogatories put to the Sorcerers of Longni, in the presence of Adrien de Fer, Lieutenant General of Laon. These sorcerers were condemned to be burnt at the stake, for having commerce with incubi. He mentions Marguerite Bremond, who avowed that she had been led off one evening, by her own mother, to a reunion of Demons, and "found in this place six devils in human shape, but hideous to behold. After the demon dance was finished, the devils returned to the couches with the girls, and one cohabited with her for the space of half an hour, but she escaped conception, as he was seedless."

One of the distinctive characters of demons, was their infectious stink, which exhaled from all portions of the body. This odor attributed to the Devil was an hallucination to the sense of smell which entered, like those of the genesic sense, into all the complex hallucinations of Demonomania.

Examples of men cohabiting with demons, are cited by many authors of the Middle Ages. Gregory of Tours has left us the record of Eparchius, Bishop of Auvergne, who cohabited with succubi.

Jerome Cardan, physician and Italian mathematician, tells of a priest who cohabited for over fifty years, with a demon disguised as a woman.

Pic de Mirandolle, relates how another priest had commerce for over forty years with a beautiful succubus, whom he called Hermione. Bodin recounts the story of Edeline, the Prior of a religious community in Sorbonne. An adversary of Demonomaniacal doctrines, Edeline was accused by the theologians of defending demons. Before the Tribunal the Prior declared that he had been visited by Satan, in the form of a black ram, and had prostituted his body to an incubus, and only obeyed his master in preaching that sorcery was a chimerical invention. "Although the proof furnished by the registers of the Tribunal of Poitiers," remarks Calmeil, "leaves no doubt as to the alienation of the intellectual faculties at the moment of his trial, Edeline was none the less condemned to perpetual seclusion from the world."

As another striking example of hallucination, bearing upon this question of incubism, Guibert de Nogent tells of a monk, "who was sick, and retained the services of a Jew doctor. In exchange for health, the aforesaid physician, demanded a sacrifice. 'What sacrifice?' asked the monk. 'The sacrifice of that which is the most precious to men,' answered the Jew. 'What may that be?' inquired the monk. And the demon, for it was the Devil disguised as a doctor, had the audacity to explain. 'Oh curses! Oh shame! to require such a thing of a priest'—but the victim, nevertheless, did what was asked. It was the denial of Christ and the true faith."

Like psycho-sensorial hallucinations of the other senses, that of the genesic sense may assume the erotic type of disease, and is due undoubtedly, in some men, to a repletion of the spermatic vesicules. It is this that Saint Andre, physician in ordinary to Louis XIV., gives as an explanation of incubism. "The incubus,"[71] says this writer, "a chimera that had for its foundation only a dream, an over excited imagination, too often a longing after women; artifice had no less a part in the creation of the incubus,—a woman, a girl, only a devotee in name, already long before debauched, but desiring to appear virtuous to hide her crime, passes off the offenses of some lover as the act of a demon; this is the ordinary explanation. In this artifice the woman is often aided by the *suggestions* of the man—a man who has heard *succubi* speaking to him in his sleep, usually sees most beautiful women in his dreams, which, under such circumstances, are often erotic."

It is certain that an ardent imagination and exaggerated sexual appetite have played a leading *role* in the history of *incubi*, but, meantime, there may be exceptions.

Nicholas Remy, Inquisitor of Lorraine, has given a description of *impurities* committed between demons and sorcerers, according to the testimony given by those *possessed*.[72] Fortunately, he has only given a Latin version of what they have told him. He states: "*Hic igitur, sive vir incubet, sive succubet fœmina, liberum in utroque naturæ debet esse officium, nihilque omnino intercedere quod id vel minimum moretur atque impediat, si pudor, metus, horror, sensusque, aliquis acrior ingruit; il icet ad irritum redeunt omnia e lumbis affœaque prorsus sit natura.*"

Then comes the sentence of the four girls of Vosges, according to the confessions, who were named Nanette, Claudine, Nicola, and Didace, and of whom Nicholas Remy, fortunately for the masses of the profession, only speaks in Latin, lest modesty be shocked at the narration. "*Alexia Drigæa recensuit doémoni suo pœnem, cum surrigebat tentum semper extitisse quanti essent subices focarii, quos tum forte præsentes digito demonstrabat; scroto ac coleis nullis inde pendentibus*, etc." (We forbear from further quotation and for fuller particulars refer the reader to the original.)

Were these girls attacked by a malady, a complex hallucination of the senses that led them to firmly believe they were possessed or owned by a supernatural being who obliged them to abdicate their free will in his favor? Were they only, after all, prostitutes suffering from nymphomania? We can only insist that prostitution, or a low standard of morality, enters largely into the history of those *possessed* by incubi.

Aside from imaginary *vigils* (Sabbat), supposed to be frequented by those who were really insane, it is well to remember there were numerous houses of prostitution, conducted by old bawds and unscrupulous panderers, where nightly orgies occurred and scenes of wild debauchery were common. The real sorcerers boasted of their magic and their relations with demons, but, in reality, they knew nothing except the art of compounding stupefying drugs, of which they made every possible use. Having passed their entire lives in vice, their passions, instead of becoming extinct, were exalted by age. "Before ever becoming sorcerers," remarks Professor Thomas Erastus, "these *lamia* (magicians) were libidinous and in close relation with the Evil One."[73]

Pierre Dufour, the celebrated bibliomaniac, made a very lengthy and learned investigation as to the connection of sorcery with the social evil, and reaped a veritable harvest of facts, duly authenticated by the histories of trials for the crime of Demonidolatry, arriving at the conclusion that sorcery made fewer dupes than victims. Says Dufour: "Aside from a very small number of credulous magicians and sorcerers, all who were initiated in the mysteries served, or made others serve, in the abominable commerce of debauchery. The *vigil* offered a fine opportunity as a spot for such turpitudes. Such reunions of hideous companies of libertines and prostitutes was for the profit of certain knaves, and the sorcerers' assemblage was patronized by many misguided young women, who fell from grace through libidinous fascination."

Meantime, sorcery persisted always, notwithstanding judgments and executions. In the year 1574, on the denunciation of an old demented hag, eighty peasants were burned alive at Valery, in Savoy. Three years later nearly four hundred inhabitants of Haut-Languedoc perished for the same offense. In 1582 an immense number of so-called sorcerers were executed at Avignon. From 1580 to 1595 nine hundred persons accused of witchcraft were put to death.

In 1609, in the country of Labourde (Basses Pyrenees), the prisons were overcrowded with men, women and children accused of sorcery. Fires for stake-burnt victims lit up all the villages in the Province, and the courts spared no one. Many of these unfortunates accused themselves of believing in the demons of sorcery and having visited diabolical gatherings (*vigils*), where they had prostituted themselves to incubi. Others, to whom the death penalty was meted out, were innocent persons who had been *informed against*, but these, too, although denying all charges, were condemned to be burnt alive.

The same year some of the inhabitants of the country of Labourde, who had sought refuge in Spain, were accused of having carried demons into Navarre. Five of these unfortunates were burnt at the stake by order of the Inquisition, one woman being strangled and burned after her death. Even bodies were exhumed to be given to the flames. Eighteen persons were permitted to make penance for their alleged sorceries.

During two years, 1615 and 1616, twenty cases of Demonidolatry were punished in Sologne and Berry; these persons were accused of being at a vigil, without having been anointed with frictions however. An old villain, aged seventy-seven years, named Nevillon, pretended to have seen a procession of six hundred people, in which Satan took the shape of a ram, or buck, and paid the sorcerers eight sous, for the murder of a man, and five sous for the murder of a woman. They accused him of having killed animals by the aid of his bewitchings. Nevillon was hung along with those he accused. Another peasant, by the name of Gentil Leclercq, avowed that he was the son of a sorcerer, that he had been baptized at the *vigil*, by a demon called *Aspic*; he was condemned to be hanged, and his body was burnt. The same it was in the case of a man called Mainguet and his wife, together with one Antoinette Brenichon, who asserted they had all three visited a witch reunion in company.

An accusation of anthropophagy was launched against the inhabitants of Germany, by Innocent VIII., in 1484, and a hundred women were also accused of having committed murders, and cohabiting with demons.

The Inquisitors inspired the story of Nider, on the Sorceries of the Vaudois. They found, according to the testimony of certain witnesses, that these Vaudois cut the throats of their infants, in order to make magical philters, which would permit them to traverse space to attend the *vigil* of the witches, (*Sorcerers*). Other persons *accused themselves* of cohabiting with demons; some pretended they had caused disasters, floods and tempests, by the influence they had through Satan. Many submitted to the most horrible tortures with an insensibility so complete, that the theologians concluded that the fat of the first born males procured this demonological faculty for bearing pain. This general anæsthesia permits us to affirm that these unfortunates were neuropathic.

It would be a difficult matter to establish the exact number of victims offered up to the fanaticism of the Inquisition. Already, in 1436, the inhabitants in the country of Vaud, Switzerland, had been accused of anthropophagy, of eating their own children, in order to satisfy their ferocious appetites. Some one said they had submitted to the Devil, and raised the outcry that they had eaten thirteen persons within a very short time. Immediately the Judge and the Prosecutor of Eude, investigated the story. Failing to obtain the proof of eye witnesses, they subjected, according to Calmeil, hundreds of unfortunates to the tortures of the rack, after which a certain number were burned at the stake. Entire families overpowered by terror, fled from home, and found refuge in more hospitable lands; but fanaticism and death followed them like a plague.[74]

The moral and physical torture, undergone by those who were suspected of this anthropophagical sorcery, made some of the victims confess that they had the power to kill infants, by uttering charm words, and that ointments made of baby fat gave them the power to fly through the air at pleasure; that the practice of Demonic science permitted them to cause cows and sheep to abort, and, that they could make thunder and hail storms, and destroy the crops of others; that they could create flood and pestilence, etc. This was the anthropophagical epidemic of 1436.

The same observations might be made regarding what was known as lycanthrophy, which always arose among the possessed and sorcerers; that is to say crazy people, especially those of the monomaniac type, accused themselves and others with imaginary crimes, in confessions made to judges. As an example, we can cite the case of the peasant, spoken of by Job Fincel, and also one mentioned by Pierre Burgot, of Verdun, who did not hesitate to assert themselves to be guilty of lycanthrophy. They were burned alive at Poligny, but the remains of the five women and children, whose flesh they pretended to have devoured, were never found. In order to transform themselves into wolves, they claimed to use a pomade given them by the Devil; and, while in a certain condition, they copulated with female wolves. Jean Wier has written long essays on this last case of lycomania, and thinks the malady of these two men was due to narcotics, of which they made habitual use; but Calmeil is inclined to consider, that in a general manner, lycomania is a partial delerium confined to homicidal monomaniacs. This appreciation of the case seems justified by the similar one of Gilles Garnier, who was convinced that he had killed four children, and eaten their flesh. He was condemned to be burnt at the stake at Dole, as a wehr-wolf, (*loupe garron*), and the peasants of the suburbs were authorized by the same order to kill off all men like him. But we must not conclude from this particular instance, that a general law existed on the subject.

In 1603, the Parliament of Bordeaux, thought itself liberal in admitting attenuating circumstantial evidence, in the case of a boy from Roche Chalais, named Jean Grenier, who was accused of lycanthropy, by three young peasants. In the trial, no attempt was made to find evidence, the accused confessed all that was desired, and he was sentenced to imprisonment for life, before which verdict was announced, the Court said, that having taken into consideration the age and imbecility of this patient, who was so stupid that an idiot or child of seven years would know better, it added mercy to the judgment."

He was then one of the imbeciles of the village, such as we see in asylums for insane, whose presence we rid ourselves of by isolation in charitable institutions.

At the same epoch, in the space of two years, 1598 to 1600, we can count the number of poor wretches of the Jura, whose poverty compelled them to beg nourishment, and who were almost all condemned to death as Demonidolators and lycanthropes. Ready and only too willing to leave this world, these poor people answered all questions as to accusation in the affirmative, and went to death with the greatest indifference. The infamous prosecutor, Bouget, who was sent into the Jura as a criminal agent, boasted that he had executed alone more than six hundred of these innocents.

The Inquistorial terror then reigned supreme; and it was only with extreme difficulty, at that time, that a poor idiot, named Jacques Roulet, condemned to death as a lycanthrope by the criminal Judge of Angers, was placed in an asylum for idiots, by order of the Parliament of Paris; this, too, in the seventeenth century.

THE HYSTERO-DEMONOMANIA OF THE CLOISTER.

The demonomaniacal hysteria of the Cloister, of which we have enumerated a few examples of a most remarkable kind, was present, in the Middle Ages, in the form of an epidemic neurosis, characterized by complex disturbances of the nervous system between the life of relation and of organic life; that is to say, by functional symptoms dependent on the general sensibility of the organs of sense, the active organs of movement, and the intelligence. In our observations we shall consequently recognize:

Hyperæsthesia and spasm of the stomach and abdominal organs, in the hallucination of poisoning by witches.

Hyperæsthesia of the ovary and the uterus and vagina, from the hallucination of painful cohabitation with incubi.

Spasms of the pharynx and laryngeal muscles: coughs, screams and barks of the prodromic period to convulsive attacks.

Vaso-motor disturbances, in the cutaneous marks, which are attributed to the Devil, but are simply produced by contact with some foreign body.

Somnambulism, in the execution of movements (sometimes in opposition with the laws of equilibrium), in a lucid state of mind, outside the condition of wakefulness, with or without mediumistic faculties and the conservation of memory; in the perception of sensations, without the intervention of the senses; in sensorial hallucinations produced by a simple touch; in *ecstasy*, with loss of tactile sense and hallucinations of vision.[75]

Suggestion, unconsciously provoked in rapid modifications of sensibility, in alterations of motility, in automatic movements executed in *imitation* (*one form of suggestion*), or by the domination of a foreign willpower, and, in general, *in the penetration of an idea or phenomenon into the brain*, by word, gesture, sight, or thought.[76]

Catalepsy, in the immobility of the body, the fixity of the regard, and the rigidity of the limbs in all attitudes, that we desire to place them (*a very rare* phenomenon).

Lethargy, in the depression of all parts of the body, and a predisposition on the part of the muscles to contract.

Delirium, finally, in the impossibility of hoping to discern false from true sensations.

We find, after this, that in analyzing the principal symptoms of hystero-demonomania, we easily note the characteristics of ordinary hysterical folly; we see that *it always attacks* by preference the impressionable woman. She who is fantastic, superstitious, hungry for notoriety, full of emotions,—one who possesses to the highest degree the gift of assimilation and imitation,— the subject of nightmare, nocturnal terrors, palpitations of the heart; a woman fickle in sentiment, one passing easily from joy to sadness, from chastity to lubricity,—a woman, in a word, who is capable of all manner of deceit and simulation, a natural-born deceiver.

The attacks of delirium among hystero-demonomaniacs have always a pronounced acute character; but, although violent and repeated, they are liable to disappear rapidly, and are often followed by relapse. These attacks of delirium are observed:

1. *Before the convulsive attacks*, under the form of melancholia or agitation, with hallucinations of sight and hearing.

2. *During convulsive attacks*, in the period of passional attitudes, under the most varied forms, by gestures in co-ordination with the hallucinations observed by the mind of the patient; we often see such persons express the most opposite sentiments—piety, erotism, and terror.

3. *After convulsive attacks*, in the form of despair, shame, rage, sadness, with an abundant shedding of tears.

4. *Without convulsive attacks*; in that case, the delirium may occur at any period; it is masked hysteria, which has a very great analogy to masked epilepsy.

The delirium of these patients, *en resume*, has for essential characteristics, exaltation of the intelligence, peculiar fixity of ideas, perversion of the sentiments, absence of will power, tendency to erotism. In a number of observations on delirium among hysterical cases in a state of hypnotism recently published, patients have been noted who believed that they cohabited with cats and monkeys, while some had hallucinations of phantoms and assassins—visions that resulted from complex hallucinations and have a certain similarity to those of hystero-demonomania observed in the Middle Ages; and, if the demons did not actually play the principle *role* in these hallucinations, it is because the imagination had not the anterior nourishment and belief in supernaturalism and no faith in the sexual relations of demons with mankind.

It was in 1491, about the time Jeanne Pothiere was on trial, that it was noticed that young girls in religious communities were subject to an epidemic mental affection, which led its victims to declare that they had fallen into the power of evil spirits. This species of delirium betrayed itself to the eyes of its observers by a series of strange and extravagant acts. These patients at once pretended to be able to read the future and prophesy. (See Calmeil, work cited.)

Abusive religious practices, false ideas of the future life, a tendency to mysticism, the fear of Hell and the snares of the Devil, the development of hysterical neurosis, in one subject, into suggestion inherent to imitation; such was the succinct history of the epidemic of the nuns of Cambrai. Jeanne Pothiere, their companion, denounced by them, was condemned to perpetual imprisonment, for having cohabited "434 times" (so the nuns said) with a Demon, and having introduced the lustful devil into their before peaceful convent. For it could have been nothing less than a demon that chased the poor young nuns across the fields and assisted them to climb trees, where, suspended from the branches, they were inspired to divine hidden things, to foretell the future, and be the victims of convulsions.

Sixty years later, in 1550, there suddenly occurred a great number of hystero-demonomaniacal epidemics similar to that in the convent of Cambrai. The nuns of Uvertet, following a strict fast, were attacked by divers nervous disorders. During the night they heard groans, when they burst out in peals of hysterical laughter; following this manifestation, they claimed they were lifted out of their beds by a superior force; they had, at the same time, contractions in the muscles of the limbs and of the face. They attacked each other in wild frenzy, giving and taking furious blows; at other times they were found on the ground, as though "inanimate," and to this species of lethargy succeeded a maniacal agitation of great violence. Like the nuns of Cambrai, they climbed trees and ran over the branches as agile as so many cats, descending head downwards with feet in the air. These manifestations were, of course, attributed to a compact with the Devil, and the officers of the law, acting on the accusations of these nuns, arrested a midwife residing in the neighborhood, on the charge of witchcraft (*sorcery*). It is needless to add that the midwife died soon after.

A neurosis almost similar occurred the same year among the nuns at Saint Brigette's Convent. In their attacks these nuns imitated the cries of animals and the bleating of sheep. At chapel one after the other were taken with convulsive syncope, followed by suffocation and œsophageal spasms, which sometimes persisted for the space of several days and condemned the victims to an enforced fast. This epidemic commenced after an hysterical convulsion occurred in one of the younger nuns, who had entered the convent on account of disappointment in love. Convinced that this unfortunate creature had imported a devil into the religious community, she was banished to one of the prisons of the Church.

At about this same time another epidemic of hystero-demonomania broke out at the Convent of Kintorp, near Strasbourg. These nuns insisted that they were possessed. Convulsions and muscular contractions which followed these attacks, along with delirium, were attributed to epilepsy. Progressively, and as though by contagion, all the nuns were stricken. When the hysterical attack arrived they uttered howls, like animals, then assaulted each other violently, biting with their teeth and scratching with finger-nails. Among those having convulsions the muscles of the pharynx participated in the general spasmodic condition. The attack was announced by a fetid breath and a sensation of burning at the soles of the feet. One day some of the young sisters denounced the convent cook, Elise Kame, as a sorcerer, although she suffered like the others from convulsive hysteria. This accusation finished the poor girl, who, together with her mother, was committed alive to the flames. Their death, most naturally, did not relieve the convent of the disease; the nervous malady, on the contrary, spread around in the neighborhood of the institution, attacking married women and young girls, whose imaginations were overpowered by the recital of occurrences within the convent walls.

We must admit that at that period doctors confounded hysteria with epilepsy. Spasms of the larynx, muscular contractions that we of the present day can provoke experimentally, as well as other phenomena of hysterical convulsions in somnambulic phases of hypnotism, were considered at that period only the manifest signs of diabolical possession. As to the stinking breath, which revealed the presence of the Devil among the nuns, that is a frequent symptom in grave affections of the nervous system; it is often a prodroma of an attack or series of maniacal convulsions. We have found that this fetidity of breath coincides with the nauseating odor of sweat and urine, to which we attribute the same semeological value as that of the mouth.

Another epidemic of hysterical convulsions, complicated with nymphomania, occurred at Cologne in 1554, in the Convent of Nazareth. Jean Wier, who was sent to examine these patients, recognized that the nuns were possessed by the Demon of lubricity and debauchery, who ruled this convent to a frightful extent.

P. Bodin has himself furnished the proofs; it was this author who wrote the history of erotic nuns. He remarks: "Sometimes the bestial appetites of some women lead them to believe in a demon; this occurred in the year 1566, in the Diocese of Cologne, where a dog was found which, it was claimed, was inhabited by a demon; this animal bit the religious ladies under their skirts. It was not a demon, but a natural dog. A woman who confessed to sinning with a dog was once burned at Toulouse.

"But it may be that Satan is sometimes sent by God, as certain it is that all punishment comes from him, through his means or without his means to avenge such crimes, as happened in a convent in Hesse, in Germany, where the nuns were demonomaniacs and sinned in a horrible manner with an animal."

Thus says Bodin, the public prosecutor of sorcerers among the laity and the religious orders. Would he not have shown much greater wisdom if he had humanely judged the actions of mankind, and had condemned as social absurdities the innumerable convents and monasteries to which the fanaticism of the Middle Ages attracted so many men and women who might have followed more useful avocations? The convulsions of nymphomaniac girls were very wild, and diversified by curious movements of the pelvis, while lying in a position of dorsal decubitus, with closed eyelids. After such attacks these poor nervous nuns were perfectly prostrated, and only breathed with the greatest difficulty. It was thus with young Gertrude, who was first attacked by a convulsive neurosis which it was claimed had been induced by nymphomaniac practices in the convent, and that evil spirits possessed these nuns.

In 1609, hystero-demonomania made victims in the Convent of Saint Ursula, at Aix. Two nuns were said to be *possessed*; these were Madeleine de Mandoul and Loyse Capel. They were exorcised without success. Led to the Convent of Saint Baume, they denounced Louis Gaufridi, priest of the Church of Acoules of Marseilles, as being a sorcerer, who had bewitched them.

The Inquisitor Michaelis has left us the history of this trial by exorcism. These patients had all the symptoms of convulsive hysteria, with nymphomania, catalepsy, and hallucinatory delirium. This Judge, however, only saw in these manifestations the work of several demons, who tormented these nuns one after, the other, at the instigation of the priest, Louis Gaufridi, who was arrested, tried, condemned by the executioner, and led to the gallows with a rope around his neck, in bare feet, a torch in hand; thus punished, the unfortunate and innocent priest fell into a state of dementia, and while in this condition confessed that he was the author of the nuns' demonomania.

As soon as Gaufridi had been sentenced to death by the Inquisition, the nuns of Saint Brigette's Convent, at Lille, who had assisted at the exorcism of the nuns of Saint Ursula, in turn were attacked by hystero-demonomania. The report soon spread that they, too, were possessed, and the Inquisitor Michaelis came to Avignon to exorcise the demons. One of these nuns, Marie de Sains, suspected of sorcery, was sent to jail. Three of her companions, treated by exorcism, denounced the unfortunate girl as a witch. Marie de Sains, who, up to this time, had asserted innocence, finished by declaring herself guilty towards the rest of the nuns in the cloister. The demons found under the nuns' beds were placed there, according to Marie's statement, by the unfortunate Gaufridi.

She testified that, "the Devil, to recompense the priest, gave him the title of 'Prince of Magicians;' and promised me," added the nun, "all kinds of sovereign honors for having consented to poison the other nuns' minds by witchcraft. Sister Joubert, Sister Bolonais, Sister Fournier, Sister Van der Motte, Sister Launoy, and Sister Peronne, who were first to have symptoms of *possession* through diabolical power, soon fell under the action of the potent philter. The witchcraft was made with the host and consecrated blood, powdered billy goat horns, human bones, skulls of children, hair, finger-nails, flesh, and seminal fluid from the sorcerer; by adding to this mixture pieces of the human liver, spleen, and brain, Lucifer gave to the hideous melange a virtue of terrible strength. The sorcerers who gave this horrible concoction to their acquaintances not only destroyed them, but also a large number of new-born children."

This unfortunate, besides, accused herself of having caused the death of a number of persons, including children, the mother, and often godmother; she claimed to have administered debilitating powders to many others. She confessed to casting an evil spell on the other nuns, which had given them over to lubricity; declared she had been to the witch *vigils* and cohabited with devils, and that she had also committed sodomy, had intercourse with *dogs*, *horses*, and *serpents*; finally, she acknowledged that she had accorded her favors to the priest, Louis Gaufridi, whereas the nun was really innocent.

Marie de Sains was found guilty of being possessed by a demon. She was exorcised and condemned to perpetual imprisonment and most austere penances by the Court of Tournay.

Immediately after the trial of Marie de Sains another nun, Simone Dourlet, was tried for the crime of sorcery, and by force of torture and *suggestions*, she admitted to have been at a witch *vigil* and was guilty. The history of this poor girl is revolting, for not only was she innocent of all crimes imputed to her, but she was not even sick. She was the victim of the hallucinations of her companions.

Another form of hystero- or hysterical demonomania was observed the same year near Dax, in the Parish of Amon, where more than 120 women were attacked by *impulsive insanity*, following the expression of Calmeil, but which has been designated by others as the *Mal de Laira*. This neurosis, which was only a variety of hysteria, was characterized by convulsions and loud barking. De L'Ancre gives an interesting description of this outbreak, but does not fail to attribute the affection to sorcerers. "It is a monstrous thing," says he, "to see in church more than forty persons, all braying and barking like dogs, as on nights when the moon is full. This music is renewed on the entrance of every new sorcerer, who has perhaps given the disease to some other woman. These possessed creatures commence barking from the time they enter church."

The same barking symptoms were noticed in dwellings when these witches passed along the street, and all passers by commenced to bark also when a sorcerer appeared.

The convulsions resembled those noticed in enraged insane persons. During the attack the victims would wallow on the earth, beating the ground with their bodies and limbs, turning their violence on their own persons without having will power to control their madness for evil doing. According to Calmeil their cases were rather hysterical than of an epileptic type.

A very remarkable fact in regard to this neurosis was that those women who howled were exempt from convulsions and reciprocally. These howls or barks were comparable to the cries uttered by the nuns of Kintorp and the bleatings of the sisters of Saint Brigette.

We have also the record of a German convent, where the nuns meowed like cats, and ran about the cloister imitating feline animals.

It is useless to add that the *Mal de Laira* was a cause of several condemnations of nuns who admitted they had bewitched their companions.[77]

Among the numerous trials for Demonidolatry, that which has been most noted was certainly the case of Urbain Grandier, and the Ursulines of Loudun, from 1632 to 1639.

The Convent of Loudun was founded in 1611 by a dame of Cose—Belfiel. Only noble ladies were received therein—Claire de Sazilli, the Demoiselles Barbezier, Madmoiselle de la Mothe, the Demoiselles D'Escoubleau, etc. These titled ladies had all received brilliant educations, but had submitted to life in a nunnery by vocation. Seven of these young women were suddenly attacked by hallucinations. They all claimed to be victims of witchcraft.

During the night these girls went in and out of the convent doors, sometimes standing on their heads, as is the case with certain individuals subject to natural somnambulism. These nuns all accused a chaplain of the order recently deceased of causing their troubles, and several of the ladies claimed that the chaplain's ghost made shameful propositions to them.

The disease grew worse from day to day, until Justice was called on to interfere, when the nuns changed their minds and declared that the real cause of their possession was in reality one Urbain Grandier, priest to the Church of Saint Pierre of Loudun, a man distinguished for his brilliant intelligence, perfect education, but rather given to gallantry, and a desire for public notoriety.

Was it Mignon, the new chaplain of the order, who *suggested* to the nuns their pretended persecutor?

That was the story, but Urbain Grandier attached no importance to the rumor.

The attacks of the nuns increased more and more, however, and were complicated with catalepsy, ecstasy and nymphomania, the victims making obscene and shameful remarks. Then exorcisers were called in, but met with no success. These ladies on the contrary endeavored to provoke the priests by lascivious gestures and indecent postures. Some of them wriggled over the floor like serpents, while others moved their bodies backwards so that their heads touched their heels, a motion, according to eye-witnesses, made with the most extraordinary quickness. At times the nuns screamed and howled in unison like a chorus of wild beasts.

A historian of the time, De Le Menardy, witness *de visu et de auditu*, has written: "In their contortions they were as supple and easily bent as a piece of lead— in such a way that their bodies could be bent in any form—backwards, forwards and sidewise, even so the head touched the earth, and they remained in these positions up to such a time as their attitudes might be changed." These movements were especially produced during the time of the attempted exorcisms. At the first mention of Satan "they raised up, passed their toes behind their necks, and, with legs separated, rested themselves on their perinæums and gave themselves up to indecent manual motions." They were delirious at this time from demonomanical excitement. Madam de Belfiel claimed to be sitting on seven devils, Madam de Sazilli had ten demons under her, while Sister Elizabeth modestly asserted her number of imps to be five.

During the exorcisms these poor women *fell sound asleep*, which induces Calmeil to think "the condition of these women resembled closely that of *magnetic somnambulists*." This supposition would permit us to explain the impossibility of the nuns telling on certain days what they had said or done during the course of a nervous attack. The days when they escaped *contortions*—when they were to the contrary violently exalted by the nature of these tactile and visceral sensations—they recalled too much, for the power of reflection disgusted these unfortunates with their own vile and uncontrollable acts and assertions.

This epidemic had continued fifteen months, and all the Ursuline nuns had been attacked by the epidemic when Laubardemont, one of the secret agents of the Cardinal Richelieu, arrived at Loudun to examine into the alleged Demonidolatry said to exist in the convent. The Cardinal had given this agent absolute and extended power. Urbain Grandier, who was the author of a libel against Richelieu, was arrested for complicity in this sorcery, and brought before a commission of Justices, whose members had been chosen by Laubardemont. He was confronted by the nuns, invited to exorcise them, and then subjected to most cruel tortures. Iron needle points were stuck in his skin, all over the body, in order to find anæsthetised points, which were the pretended marks of the Devil.

Notwithstanding his protestations of innocence, the Judges taking the acts of the accusers while in the poor priest's presence, for his appearance was the signal for scenes of the most violent frenzy, condemned the man to be tied to a gallows alive. There he was subjected to renewed tortures, while the various muscles of his body were torn apart and his bones broken.

The punishment of Urbain Grandier did not put an end to the epidemic of hysterical demonomania among the Ursulines, for the malady extended to the people of the town, even to the monks who were charged with conducting the exorcisms; but the vengeance of his Red Eminence (Cardinal Richelieu) was satisfied.

Many commentaries have been made since then on this outbreak of Demonidolatry among the Ursulines. These we have no desire to reproduce nor to discuss, as it would only tend to show the ancient ignorance prevailing regarding diseases of the nervous system, and the want of character and weakness of the physicians of that epoch, together with the fanaticism of the monks and priesthood. One thing, however, appears to be worthy of remembrance; that is the analogy between the convulsive symptoms observed among the nuns and the phenomena of somnambulism described by Calmeil. This fact appears to us as so much the more remarkable, as the learned doctor of Charenton was a declared adversary of magnetism, and published his work almost half a century since—that is, in 1845.

The sleep into which the nuns fell during the period of exorcism, the forgetfulness of the scenes witnessed where they had played such a *role*, are, to our mind, only phenomena of hypnotism, and the resemblance is so strong that we do not believe it would be impossible to artificially reproduce another epidemic of hysterical demonomania.

Let us for an instant accept the *hypothesis* of a convent, where twenty young nuns are confined. Of these at least ten will be subject to hypnotism. Let us now admit that these recluses, living the ordinary ascetic and virtuous life of the cloister, plunged deeply in the mysticisms of the Catholic faith, receive one day as confessor and spiritual director a man of energetic character, knowing all the practices of *hypnotism* and of *suggestion*—a disciple let us say of Puel, Charcot, De Luys, Barety, Bernheim—a perfect neurologist. Now, if this man cared to magnetize individually each of these nuns in the silence and obscurity of the confessional, and should then suggest to them that they were *possessed* by all the demons known to sorcery, what would occur? Let us suppose again that he should carry his physiological power further and put his *subjects* into an ecstacy, catalepsy or lethargy—into a condition where marked hallucinations might occur and nervous excitation be provoked, how long would it be before this man could make these women similar to those who once lived in the convent of the Ursulines at Loudun?

We have not admitted this fiction for the purpose of having any one conclude that the possessed of Loudun were the mere playthings of some person who used hypnotism in an interest that we ignore; but, if this fact may be considered possible by the will of an individual, who can affirm at this day that there does not exist an unknown force, intelligent or not, capable of producing the same pathological phenomena observed long ago? What we call, in 1888, hypnotism in the amphitheatres of our universities, we reserve for another chapter, where we will give revelations much more extraordinary, and also more supernatural; our chapter on the neurology of the nineteenth century will, we promise, be *very interesting*.

Let us yet remark that the hystero-demonomaniacal manifestations were not peculiar to the Ursulines of Loudun. They have been observed in many convents in the same conditions of habits and prolonged fastings among debilitated young girls; from long vigils spent in prayer and nervous depression, caused by over-religious discipline; by mystical exhortations from a man invested in a sacred character, on whom fall all the discussions, all the entreaties, and all the thoughts of the girls in the cloister.

The history of the nuns of Loudun was identically reproduced under the same conditions among the sisters of Saint Elizabeth's Convent at Louviers, in 1643, three years after the execution of poor Urbain Grandier for witchcraft.

In a short time eighteen nuns were attacked with hysterical demonomania; they had active hallucinations of all the senses, convulsions, and delirium. Like the Ursulines, they blasphemed, screamed, and gave themselves over to all manner of strange contortions, claiming to be *possessed* by demons, describing in obscene terms the orgies of the witch vigil (*Sabbat*), perpetrating all varieties of debauchery, even unknown to the vilest prostitutes; after this they finally accused one or more persons of bewitching them through sorcery.

The nuns of Louviers, for instance, after being duly exorcised according to the Canons of the Church, accused as the author of their affliction, and as a bad magician, their old time confessor, the Abbot Picard, who died before their symptoms were developed; then they accused another priest, by the name of Francois Boulle, and several of their companions, notably Sister Madeleine Bavan. These innocent people were tried by the Parliament of Rouen, who ordered that the body of the priest, Picard, should be exhumed, carried to the stake, there tied to the living body of Francois Boulle, and after being burnt their ashes should be cast to the winds. This execution, in the open air, occurred in the seventeenth century, in the "Old Market Place" at Rouen, at the spot where Joan d'Arc had also been burnt alive for being *possessed*, as was claimed, by supernatural beings. What a comment on intelligence in an age of partial enlightenment!

In order to close this chapter on hysterical demonomania among religious orders, of which we have given some examples, we shall cite an interesting relation left us by the Bishops and Doctors of Sorbonne, together with the testimony of the King's deputies, regarding the *possession* of nuns at the Convent of Auxonne. Here there were always convulsions and screams, with blasphemy, aversion to taking the sacraments, possession, and exorcisms; and there was, undoubtedly, the phenomenon of *suggestion* observed with much precision.

We might say that the nuns of Auxonne were accessible to suggestion; for, at the command or even the thought of the exorcists, they fell into a condition of somnambulism; in this state they became insensible to pain, as was determined by pricking Sister Denise under the finger-nail with a needle; they had also the faculty of prosternating the body, making it assume the form of a circle,—in other words, they could bend their limbs in any direction.

The Bishop of Chalons reports that "all the before mentioned girls, secular as well as regular, to the number of eighteen, *had the gift of Language*, and responded to the exorcists *in Latin*, making, at times, their entire conversation in the classical tongue.

"Almost all these nuns had a full knowledge of the secrets and inner thoughts of others;[78] this was demonstrated particularly *in the interior commandments*, which had been made by the exorcists on different occasions, which they obeyed exactly ordinarily, *without the commandments being expressed to them either by words or any external sign.*

"The Bishop himself, among others, experimented on the person of Denise Pariset, to whom, *giving a command mentally to come to him immediately and be exorcised,* whereupon the aforesaid nun immediately came to him, although her residence was in a quarter of the village far removed from the Episcopal residence. She said on these occasions that she was commanded to come; and this experiment was repeated several times.

"Again, in the person of Sister Jamin, a novice, who on hearing the exorcism, told the Bishop his interior commandment made to the Demon during the ceremony. Also, in the person of Sister Borthon, who, being *commanded mentally* to make her agitations violent, immediately prostrated herself before the Holy Sacrament, with her belly against the earth and her arms extended, executing the command at the same instant, with a promptitude and precipitation wholly extraordinary."[79]

Here, I believe, are facts so well authenticated of transmission of thought or of mental *suggestions,* perhaps *voluntarily unknown* to certain modern neurologists. These neuropaths of Auxonne presented still more extraordinary phenomena; at the word of command they suspended the pulsations of the pulse in an arm, in the right arm, for example, and transfered the beatings from the right arm to the left arm, and *vice versa.* This fact was discovered by the Bishop, and many ecclesiastics verified the same, and "it was promptly done in the presence of Doctor Morel, who recognized and makes oath to the fact."

We cannot dwell too long on the Demonomania of the Middle Ages, to which we have, perhaps, added some historical facts which are new and which we believe it to be our duty to publish, seeing a connection with modern hypnotism. We shall thus open a new field for investigation on strange affections, classed up to the present time in all varieties of monomania, but which appear to us to belong to a variety of mental pathology independent of insanity, properly speaking. If it were otherwise it would be necessary to recognize as crazy persons, not only the Demonomaniacs of the Middle Ages, but also the Jansenists, who went into trances, and the choreics and convulsionists (*convulsionnaires*) of the eighteenth century. They were certainly not crazy, those who came to the mortuary of Saint Medard, to the tomb of the Deacon Paris, to make an appeal against the Papal bull of Clement XI. And was it not another cause than auto suggestion, to which it is necessary to attribute the nervous phenomena that the *appelants* exhibited during thirty consecutive years?

The exaltation of religious ideas, so often advanced by psychologists, cannot account for these phenomena. I have seen palpable proofs of this in the various accidents that suddenly overcame sceptics and strong-minded men of modern times, who came as amateurs to assist at the experiments on convulsive subjects. These symptoms, as is well known, are usually ushered in by violent screams, rapid beatings of the heart, contractions of muscles, and analogous nervous symptoms.

Besides, it is incontestible that many patients and infirm people obtain an unhoped for cure following convulsive cries; while others, in a state of health, are taken with hallucinations and delirium. I have seen patients who would lacerate certain portions of the body that were the seat of burns, and continue to walk, cry, gesticulate, and abuse themselves, like insane persons in a real state of dementia.

The Jansenists did not speak, had no compacts with demons, no exorcisms at which Inquisitors and their acolytes could suggest ideas of demonomania; and notwithstanding their great austerities and the most rigorous fasts, we note among the *convulsionnaires* of Saint Medard only the ideas of possession by the Holy Spirit and divine favors obtained through the protection of the kind-hearted Deacon; and meantime, those possessed by God, as by the Devil, were subjects of somnambulism, to trances, lethargy, catalepsy, and other phenomena.[80]

The last analogy, finally, between the two nervous epidemics, was the Royal authority, a special form of *suggestion* in the Middle Ages, which put an end to sorcery or witchcraft as well as to Jansenism.

HYSTERIA AND PSYCHIC FORCE.

Among the phenomena observed in demonomaniacal hysteria there are some, as we have remarked, that modern neurologists have wished to *pass over in silence*, because it was impossible to give a rational explanation. It arose from that mysterious force which acts upon the human personality and its faculties and produces *supernatural results* in contradiction to well known scientific laws, known in one sense as *Psychic Force*, but which is nothing else than *modern spiritualism*.

This force, a power possessed in a high degree not only by hysterical persons, but all varieties of neuropaths, who are designated as *mediums* by spiritual psychologists, *cannot be doubted by real scientists to day.*

The demonologists of the Middle Ages have often mentioned it in the demonomaniacs, and attributed it to possession by evil spirits; and, if not pathologists, *they did not disdain to occupy themselves with something that tends to simplify the study of the physiology of the nervous system*; but to minds of the modern type, that consider science as synonymous with truth, it seems strange and incomprehensible that our learned investigators should have been overpowered by the fear of the criticism that might overtake them because *they cannot explain purely and simply an inexplicable fact, a truth, real positive and certain.*

Not being ourselves timorous to this prudence, which is, they claim, one of the conditions, *sine qua non*, to be a candidate for the Institute of France, we shall now pursue our investigations with the historical documents regarding the medical Middle Age we possess, and thus loyally seek a scientific interpretation for facts observed in modern spiritualism or *psychic force*.

Among these documents we will choose as a type the "Trial made to deliver a girl possessed by the Evil Spirit, at Louviers." This suit, which dates back to 1591, is in reality a series of trials written up by several magistrates, in the presence of numerous witnesses, reporting with precision all facts observed by them—facts interpreted, it is true, with ideas of the demonidolatry of the sixteenth century, but having a character whose authenticity is undisputed, and *even undiscussed.* The first trial is thus conceived:[81]

"On Saturday, the 18th day of August, 1591, in the morning at Louviers, in the aforesaid place, before us, Louis Morel, Councillor of the King, Provost General and Marshal of France for the Province of Normandy, holding Court in the service of the King in the villages and castles of Pont de l'Arche and Louviers, with one lieutenant, one recorder, and fifty archers, assisted by Monsieur Behotte, licentiate of law, Judge Advocate and Lieutenant General of Monsieur the Viscount of Rouen, in the presence of Louis Vauquet, our clerk." * * *

This old document, in French now almost obsolete and difficult of translation,[82] goes on to state that in a house at Louviers, belonging to Mrs. Gay, two officers, belonging to the troops occupying the town, who had temporary quarters with Gay, complained to their commandant that "a spirit in the house mentioned tormented them." Now, this house was occupied by three ladies: Madame Gay, one of her friends, a widow named Deshayes, and a servant girl called Francoise Fontaine.

Captain Diacre, who was commandant of the village, found on investigation the general disorder of the residence, the furniture turned upside down, the two ladies terrified, and the servant girl with several wounds on her body. The latter was suspected of being in league with the Devil, and was arrested and cast into the prison of the town. On her person was found a purse containing a teston (old French coin), a half teston, and a ten-sous piece. The trial proved nothing. The ladies might have had nightmare, the officers might have been drunk, the noises heard might have been the result of a thousand different causes, but it is necessary to mention this case in order to comprehend the subsequent trials.

The second trial, witnessed, tried, and authenticated by the same authorities, determined the fact that Francoise Fontaine was born at Paris, Faubourg Saint Honore, and that at the age of twenty two years she had already witnessed similar phenomena in a house "haunted," said she, "by evil spirits that frightened her so much that she went to a neighbor's to sleep while her mistress was absent from home." This statement was proved correct in six subsequent trials containing the depositions of Marguerite Prevost, Suzanne Le Chevalier, Marguerite Le Chevalier, and Perrine Fayel.

The following trial states that on Saturday, the 31st of August, 1591, before Louis Morel, Councillor of the King, assisted by his clerk, Louis Vauquet, etc., etc.,

"Came Pierre Alix, first jailer and guard of the prison, who threw himself on his two knees before us, holding the prison keys in his hand, pale and overcome by emotion; for which action we remonstrated, when he stated to our great astonishment that he did not wish to longer act as prison guard, for the reason that the evil spirit that tormented the aforesaid Francoise Fontaine likewise tormented him, and also the prisoners, who desired to break jail and fly in order to save themselves, having a presentement that the aforesaid Francoise Fontaine, was in a dungeon or pit, and *that she had removed a great iron door that had fallen upon her afterwards*; and several persons having ran to her along with the jailer found the aforesaid Fontaine acting as though possessed by an evil spirit, with her throat swollen," etc.

Let us pass over an interminable recital made by Francoise Fontaine to the priests and counsellors of the King, relative to *diabolic possession*, to which she had been subject all her life. Also, as to the testimony of many witnesses as to her performance while in jail; as, for instance, "the body of Francoise rose in the air about four feet, without being in contact with anything, and she floated towards us in the air," etc., etc.

Francois Fontaine claimed that she had consented to belong to the Demon, who was "a black man with whom she had cohabited." Considered from a medical standpoint the girl was a victim to hysterical demonomania.

Let us make a few more extracts from the records of this trial:

"As the aforesaid Fontaine told us these things, being meantime on her two knees before us, who were seated on a raised platform, the aforesaid Fontaine fell forward on her face as though she had been struck from above, and the candles in the chandeliers of the room were extinguished, except those on the clerk's table, the which were roughly blown upon several times without being put out, when no visible person present was near them to blow, and these candles were raised out of their candlesticks, lighted as they were, and rubbed against the ground in an attempt to extinguish them, and the which were finally extinguished with a great noise, without any human hand appearing near them; the which so astonished the priest, the advocate, the first jailer, the archers guard, who were present, that they retired, leaving us alone, the hour being then nine o'clock at night.

"Finding myself alone, I recommended my soul to God, and exclaimed in a loud voice the words, 'My God, give me grace not to lose my soul to the Devil, and I command thee O, Demon, by the power I have invoked, to leave the body of Francoise Fontaine! Again I repeat the command!'"

At the same instant the exorcist felt himself seized by the legs, arms and body, and tightly held in the arms of an unknown force, which felt hot and blew a warm breath, while blows were rained on the Judge's body as though he were beaten by a heavy piece of wood. He was struck on the jaw and under the ear hard enough to draw blood, etc.

At the eleventh trial it was found that Francoise Fontaine was bodily raised out of bed during the night by an unseen force, and this fact is duly authenticated by witnesses.

In the following trial the same phenomena were produced in the church at Louviers, during the mass of exorcism, where:

"Francoise Fontaine floated from the earth into the air, higher than the altar, as though lifted up by the hair by an unseen hand, which quickly alarmed the assistants, who had never before witnessed such an occurrence," etc.

In presence of these facts Francoise was led back to prison, and it was decided by the clerical council, assisted by two eminent physicians, Roussel and Gautier, to cut off the girl's hair, as was the custom when witches were arrested.

During this operation, which was performed publically by Dr. Gautier, the same phenomenon was reproduced. For says the veracious old French chronicle: "Francoise est de rechef enleuee en l'air fort hault, la tete en bas, les pieds en hault sans que ses accoustrementz se soient renuersez, au trauers desquelz il sortoit par deuant et par derriere grande quantite d'eaue et fumee puante."

Like the many preceding trials, with experiments, which are duly attested by magistrates, physicians and the clerk, seven person in all, who witnessed the phenomena, as to material facts, we cannot suspect people whose honesty was never doubted; for it was through their influence that Francoise Fontaine was set at liberty, after all her inexplicable symptoms had disappeared and her nervous malady abated.

In order to render an account of the *supernatural* phenomena observed by early demonographers and attributed to evil spirits, let us briefly glance at the experiments made regarding *Spiritualism* by a few brave physiologists of our own epoch, who have dared to investigate the analogy existing between these two orders of phenomena.

Among the modern experimenters who have made a scientific study of this subject—let us call it *Psychic Force*, if you will—we will mention Mr. Crookes, member of the Royal Society of London, the (English Academy of Sciences), the master mind, the most illustrious in modern science; the discoverer of thallium, radiant matter, photometer of polarization, spectral microscope— a chemist and physicist of the first order, accustomed to the most minute experimental investigations.

The experiments of this *savant* have been arranged by him in three classes, as follows:

CLASS I.—*Movement of weighty bodies with contact, but without mechanical effort.*

This movement is one of the most simple forms of the phenomenon observed; it presents degrees that vary from trembling or vibration of the chamber and its contents up to the complete elevation in the air, when the hand is placed above, of a weighty body. We commonly object that when they touch an object put in motion, they push, draw or raise it. I have experimentally proved that this is impossible in a great number of cases; but, as a matter of evidence, I attach little importance to that class of phenomena considered in themselves, and have only mentioned them as a preliminary to other movements of the same kind, but without contact.

"These movements (and I may truly add all other similar phenomena) are generally preceded by a particular breeziness of the air, amounting sometimes almost to a true wind. This air disperses leaves of paper and lowers the thermometer several degrees.

"Under some circumstances, to the subject of which I shall, at some future day, give more details, I have not found any of this air; but the cold was so intense that I can only compare it to that experienced by placing the hand at a short distance from mercury in a state of congelation." (*Crookes*).

I have obtained, like the eminent "member of the Royal Society of London," the movement of weighty bodies by contact very easily, not only lifting massive tables of a weight altogether out of proportion and far superior to the force of a very robust man, but have also seen this furniture move in a given direction; I have even noted a small square table keep time in beating with a determined cadence. This phenomenon, well known to all experimenters, may be reproduced without the assistance of a powerful medium; it was well known in times of antiquity, but is not mentioned in the writings on sorcery during the Middle Ages.

As extraordinary as these facts seem, they are no more singular than those observed by W. Crookes, and very recently by Zoellner,[83] Professor in the University of Leipsic and correspondent of the French Institute, in presence of Professors Fechner, Braune, Weber, Scheibner, and the celebrated surgeon, Thiersch. It was with Slade, an American medium as extraordinary as Home, that Zoellner experimented. These experiments may be thus briefly mentioned:

1. Movements made by psychic force, through the medium of Slade, of a magnet enclosed in a compass box.

2. Blows struck on a table, a knife raised in air, without contact, to the height of a foot.

3. Movement of heavy bodies. Zoellner's bed was drawn two feet from the wall, Slade remaining seated with his back to the bed, his legs covered and in full view of the experimenters.

4. A fire-screen broken with noise, without contact with the medium, and the fragments thrown five feet.

5. Writing produced on several experimental occasions between two slates belonging to Zoellner, and held well in view.

6. Magnetization of a steel needle.

7. Acid reaction given to neutral substances.

8. Imprints of hands and naked feet on smoked surfaces or surfaces powdered with flour, which did not correspond with the hands and feet of the medium, who remained meantime in full view of the experimenters, while Slade's feet were covered with shoes.

9. Knots tied in bands of copper sealed at both ends and held in the hands of Slade and Zoellner, etc.

We find the same tests and facts observed by Mr. Crookes and the French experimenters, who, following his example, have sought to account for *Psychic Force.*

CLASS II.—*Phenomenon of percussion and other analogous noises.*

The popular name of *spiritual rapping* gives a very poor idea of this class of phenomena. On different occasions during his experiments, Mr. Crookes heard blows of a delicate variety, such as might be produced by the point of a needle; a cascade of sounds, as acute as those coming from an induction coil in full activity; sharp blows or detonations in the air; acute notes of a metallic variety; rasping sounds similar to that heard from a machine with rubbing action; noises like scratching; twittering chirps like a bird, etc.

"I have observed these noises," says Crookes, "with the majority of mediums, each of whom has a special peculiarity. They were more varied with Mr. Home; but, for force and certainty of result, I have never met a medium who approached Kate Fox. For several months I experimented, it may be said, in an unlimited manner, and verified the different manifestations induced by the presence of this lady, and I especially examined the phenomenon relative to these noises.

"With mediums, it is necessary in general that they be methodically seated for the *seance* before noises are heard, but with Miss Kate Fox it was sufficient to merely place her hand on any object, no matter what, and violent blows were heard, like a triple sound of beating, and sometimes so loud as to be heard at different pieces of furniture in the room.

"In this manner, I have heard these noises on a living tree, on a fragment of glass, on a membrane extended in a frame—for instance, a tambourine—on the top of a cab, and on the edge of the parquet railing in the theatre.

"However, effective contact is not always necessary. I have heard the noise sound inside walls, when the hands and feet of the medium were tightly held; when Miss Fox was seated in a chair; when she was suspended above the platform; finally, when she had fallen on a sofa in a dead faint.

"I have heard these same noises on the harmonica; I have felt them on my shoulder and under my hands; I have heard them on a leaf of paper held between the fingers by the aid of a wire passed through one corner.

"With a perfect knowledge of the numerous theories advanced, in America principally, to explain these knocks or spirit rapping, I have verified them by all methods I could imagine, so that I have acquired a positive conviction as their objective reality, and the absolute certainty that it was impossible to produce these sounds by artifice or some mechanical means.

"An important question is here asked that deserves attention, *i.e.* '*are these noises governed by an intelligence?*'[84]

"From the commencement of my investigations, I have recognized the fact that the power which produced the phenomena, was not simply a fluid force, but that *it is associated with an intelligence, or follows its directions.*"

During the three years that I have experimented in psychology with Dr. Puel and his friends, there has been no *seance* where we have not been able to determine more or less important phenomena of percussion. An experiment I love to make is that of striking my fingers on the table, either to imitate the music of a band with drum accompaniment with some known air, and the same sound is immediately produced on the under surface of the piece of furniture, with the same rhythm appearing to be invoked by an invisible hand performing under the table. This phenomenon is manifested sometimes spontaneously upon my demand or that of my assistant. I observed it one evening at my own house for more than a quarter of an hour from, the moment I entered the room; in this case the noise was a rolling, which appeared to arise from the metallic surface of a table. It was a member of my family who called my attention to the abnormal noise, so much the more curious, inasmuch as I could produce it at will, giving shades and variations expressed by the movements of my hand. In order to respond in advance to any objection, I will say it was two o'clock in the morning when this phenomenon was produced, and there was no passing carriages in the street to make any kind of a vibration.

These phenomena of percussion are sometimes produced with a most extraordinary intensity, as in the observations of Kate Fox in the house at Hydesville; these were probably only phenomena of percussion similar to those observed at Louviers, in the home of Madame Gay, under the mediumship of Francoise Fontaine, in 1591, manifestations which were then attributed to the Devil, or later to a condition of hallucinations, among the witnesses, according to the *materialistic psychologists* of the nineteenth century.

CLASS III.—*Alteration of the weight of bodies.*

The experiments made by Mr. Crookes, in regard to the alterations in the weight of bodies, enters the category of psychic phenomena examined with the most mathematical exactitude, by the aid of accurate registering apparatus. It is in these experiments that the celebrated English physician was able to witness *Psychic Force* developed by his *medium.*

The description and designs of the apparatus thus used may be found in the *"Moniteur de la Policlinique,"* of the 7th and 14th of May, 1882, and in *"Le Spiritisme"* of Dr. Paul Gibier, published in the year 1887.

This article is too lengthy for reproduction in this work, but we have the right to consider it as the point of departure for experimental psychology, for not only have they not been denied in France and other countries, but *they have been recognized as absolutely true,* by several colleagues of Mr. Crookes, belonging to the *Royal Society of London.*

CLASS IV.—*Movements of heavy bodies at a distance from the medium.*

"There are numerous instances in which heavy objects, such as tables, chairs, ropes, etc., have been moved when the medium never touched them. I will mention a few striking cases.

"My own chair turned half way around while my feet were on the floor.

"In full view of all the people present, a chair started from a far off corner and advanced slowly to a table while we were watching its movement.

"On another occasion an arm chair came from to the place we were seated, and then, on my demand, slowly returned backward a distance of three feet.

"During three consecutive *seances*, a small table crossed the room under conditions I had especially fixed in advance, in order to respond victoriously to all objections that might possibly be raised against the reality of the phenomenon.

"I repeated on several occasions the experiment considered as conclusive by the *"Dialectic Society,"* that is to say, the movement of a heavy table in a full glare of light, the backs of chairs being turned towards the table about one foot of distance, each person being in a kneeling posture upon his chair, the hands placed upon the back above the table, but not touching it.

"On one of these occasions, the experiment took place while I walked all around the table in order to see how each person was placed." (*Crookes*).

In our own seances, with Madam Rosine, L.B., we have seen, ten or twelve times at least, a small table on rollers, advance towards us as though moved by a force of attraction or repulsion.

A similar phenomenon was very often produced in my office, under the mediumistic influences of M. D. with a strength of extraordinary propulsion, which seemed to originate in brute force. The traces of violent shocks of a table against my bureau still remain to testify to the results of this occurrence.

CLASS V.—*Chairs and tables raised from the earth without contact with any person.*

"A remark usually made when cases of this kind arise is: 'Why do these things only occur with chairs and tables? Is this a privilege solely enjoyed by pieces of furniture?' I wish to answer this by stating that I simply observed facts and report them without pretending to enter into the *why* and *how*; but, in truth, it is very evident that if any inanimate object of a certain weight can be lifted from the earth in the ordinary dining room, it could as easily be anything else than a chair or table.

"That such phenomena are not limited to furniture I have numerous proofs, as have other experimenters; the *intelligence* or *force*, whichever it may be, that produces the manifestations, can only operate with materials that are at its disposition.

"On five distinct occasions a heavy dining table was raised from the floor for a height varying from some inches to a foot and a half, under special imposed conditions that made fraud impossible.

"On another occasion a heavy table was raised to the ceiling, in full light, *while I held the feet and hands of the medium.*

"At another time the table raised itself above the floor, without any one touching it, but under conditions I had previously imposed in such a manner as to render the proof of the fact incontestable." (*Crookes.*)

The phenomena observed in this class of experiments belong to those of *movement without contact.* Although these are difficult to obtain, I have noticed them several times; I have seen, in my own home, a massive table raised some distance from the floor ten or fifteen seconds after all contact had ceased. Dr. Gibier had the advantage of obtaining complete levitation and seeing the table *turn and touch the ceiling with its four feet,* under the mediumistic influence of Mr. Slade. The Doctor affirms this fact in his own book on the subject.

In the trial of August 31st, 1591, a phenomenon similar to the one narrated befell Francoise Fontaine, *i.e.,* the fall of an iron door on the unfortunate girl; the elevation in the air of a washtub and its being emptied in the presence of the jailer and the prisoner Aufrenille. Francois Fontaine was evidently a *medium* with *psychic effects.*

CLASS VI.—*Raising human beings in the air.*

"This phenomenon has taken place in my presence four times, although in obscurity. The conditions under which these movements were performed, however, were completely satisfactory; but the ocular demonstration of such a thing is necessary to prevent the effects of our preconceived opinions; for example, upon that which is *naturally possible or impossible,* I shall only mention here cases in which the deductions of reason have been affirmed by the sense of vision.

"I saw, one day, in the quality of spectator, a chair on which a lady was seated raised from the floor several inches.

"On another occasion, in order to avoid being suspected of producing the phenomenon by artificial means, the lady knelt on the chair, so that the four legs of the piece of furniture were visible to every eye; then the chair was lifted from the floor three inches, remaining suspended in the air for ten seconds, when it slowly descended to the floor again.

"Another time, but separately, two children were raised to the ceiling in their chairs, under a full glare of light, under conditions entirely satisfactory to me, for I was on my knees and attentively watched the feet of the chairs in order to see that no one touched them.

"The most remarkable examples of levitation I have observed have taken place with Mr. Home. On three occasions I have seen him lifted to the ceiling of the room. On the first occasion he was seated in a chair, the second time he was kneeling on a chair, and the third experiment he stood on the chair. In all these instances I had every facility for examining the phenomena at the moment they occurred.

"Over a hundred instances where Mr. Home was raised from the floor in the presence of numerous witnesses have been published, and I have had the oral testimony of at least three witnesses to these exhibitions, *i.e.*, Count Dunraven, Lord Lindsay, and Captain Wynne.

"To reject the numerous depositions presented on this subject would be to reject all human testimony on any other subject; for there are no facts in history, be they sacred or profane, that are supported on such a solid basis of proof.

"The number of witnesses who will testify to the levitations of Mr. Home is overwhelming. It is to be greatly desired that persons whose testimony would be accepted as conclusive by the scientific world would seriously examine with patience these facts.

"The majority of ocular witnesses of these phenomena are still living, and will most assuredly bear witness; but in a few years it will be difficult, if not impossible, to obtain such *direct evidence* as in the case of Home." (*Crookes.*)

It is to this class of phenomena that the case of Francois Fontaine belongs, the authenticated facts of which, officially recorded and witnessed, are matters of history; her levitations in the prison at Louviers cannot be doubted.

The cataleptic symptoms accompanying the ascentional movements of this woman bear witness as to the special neuropathic condition in which she was found—a condition to-day in which most mediums develop *psychic force*, either spontaneously or following hypnotic maneuvers.

One of the benefits to future science will be the explanation given to these phenomena now considered supernatural; things that our learned Academicians refuse to believe in, *although not investigating*, insisting that such phenomena are hallucinations, the mere assertions of writers and those who witness them; while these so-called *savants*, who laugh spiritualism to scorn, claiming it a fraud and imposture, are themselves afraid to be convinced by scientific experimentation.[85]

CLASS VII.—*Movement of small objects without personal contact.*

"Under this title I propose to describe certain particular phenomena of which I have been a witness.

"I shall content myself to here allude to some facts all the more surprising, since those who have witnessed them did so under circumstances that rendered all deception impossible; it would be foolish to attribute these results to fraud, for the phenomena were not observed in the house of a medium, but in my own home, where any previous preparation was out of the question.

"A medium was taken to my dressing room and seated in a certain portion of the chamber under the watchful eyes of a number of attentive witnesses, and played an accordion *I held in my own hand* with the keys upside down; this same accordion then floated in the air, playing as it remained suspended.

"This medium could not secretly introduce to my home a machine strong enough to rattle my windows and remove Venetian blinds to the distance of eight feet; to tie knots in my handkerchief and carry it to a far-off corner of a large room; to play notes on a piano at a distance; to make a plate float around the room; to raise a water carafe from a table; to make a coral necklace stand up on one of its limber extremities; to put a fan in the usual society motions; or to start the pendulum of a clock when the time piece was sealed in glass and screwed tightly to the wall." (*Crookes.*)

These same phenomena are produced by Fakirs. A certain number of fig or other leaves are perforated by bamboo sticks stuck in the ground. The charmer extends his hands, the leaves move up along the long sticks on which they are strung.

Another experiment: a vase is filled with water and spontaneously moves over a table, leans, oscillates, is raised a perceptible height, without a drop of water being spilled.

Musical instruments render sounds, play melodious airs, under the eyes of the investigator, at some distance from the Fakir and without the latter making any apparent movement. Dr. Gibier cites these phenomena, witnessed by persons entitled to every confidence.

During seances at the home of my friend Dr. Fuel, with Madam L. B., we have witnessed similar phenomena. Several times my *confrere* and I have seen damask curtains at his office windows shake and open; have heard the sound of a small trumpet placed in the center of a table, in the dark, it is true, but we were holding each other's hands in the circle and used all possible precautions not to be duped or humbugged.

CLASS VIII.—*Luminous apparitions.*

"These manifestations are weak and generally require a darkened room. I wish to recall to my readers the fact that on these occasions I have taken all the necessary precautions to avoid being deceived by light due to luminous oils (of which phosphorous might form the basis) or other means. Besides, I have endeavored in vain to imitate these lights artificially.

"I have seen under experimental conditions of the most severe sort, a solid body having its own light about the size of a goose egg float around the room without noise at a height not to be touched even by standing on ones toes, afterwards softly descend to the floor.

"This luminous globe remained visible for more than ten minutes before disappearing; it struck the table on three occasions, making the noise produced by any hard and solid body of the same size.

"During this time, the medium was seated in an arm chair, in an apparent condition of insensibility.

"I have seen luminous sparks disport themselves above the heads of various persons.

"I have obtained response to questions by means of flashes of light, any number of times in front of my own face.

"I have seen sparks of light rise from the table and to the ceiling and fall back on the table with a distinct noise of solidity.

"I have obtained, alphabetically, a communication, by means of flashes of light, produced in mid air, before my eyes, while my hand moved around in the rays of the communicating light; I have seen a luminous cloud float up and rest on a picture.

"On several occasions, under similar conditions of severe control, a body solid in appearance but crystalline, having a light of its own, has been placed in my hand by a hand not belonging to any person present in the room. In *the full glare of light*, I have seen a luminous body fly to the top of a heliotrope placed on top of a *console*, break off a small branch of the plant and carry it to the hand of a lady present.

"I have sometimes seen similar luminous clouds *visibly condense, assume the form of a hand*, and carry small articles to people, but these phenomena properly belong to another class of manifestations." (*Crookes*).

The only phenomena of this nature that I have noticed were produced under the following circumstances: One evening, after commencing some experiments with Madam L. B., in the parlor of Dr. Puel, we were obliged to cut the *seance* short owing to a convulsive hysterical attack that overcame the medium—an attack which lasted more than an hour and which was only stopped by the application of metallic plates to the thorax. Having regained consciousness, the lady, with her husband and Dr. Puel, retired to the latter's consultation office, where I was summoned a few moments later by my *confrere*. Madam L. B. was standing, supported by my two friends,[86] while from her chest arose phosphorescent vapors, which grew more dense and thick as the lights in the room were turned down. These phenomena lasted more than a quarter of an hour, during which Madam L. B. uttered long and painful groans. These vapors had the odor of phosphorus, and seemed to rise from the epigastric region.

I was called some months later to attend to Madam L. B., whom I found in a condition of profound anæmia and mental prostration, reminding me of the *seance*; I prescribed granules of phosphoric acid for her with excellent results.

CLASS IX.—*Apparition of hands, either luminous or visible under ordinary light.*

"One finds himself frequently touched by hands, or something having the form of hands, during *dark seances*, or under circumstances which do not permit us to see these forms; but *I have seen these hands.*

"I shall not speak here of instances in which the phenomenon occurred in obscurity, but will simply choose some of the *numerous instances* in which I have seen the hands *in the light.*

"A small hand, of charming shape, has risen from the table and extended me a flower; this hand appeared and disappeared three times at intervals and gave me every opportunity to convince myself that it was, in appearance, as real as my own. This occurred in a full light, in my own room, while I held the hands and feet of the medium.

"On another occasion, a small hand and arm, similar to those of a child, appeared to play around a lady seated near me; this arm floated to my side, struck my arm lightly and pulled my coat several times.

"Another time, I saw an arm and hand tear the petals from a flower placed in Mr. Home's *boutonniere* and hold the same before the faces of parties sitting near him.

"On this occasion, and with other witnesses, who saw the same manifestations, a hand touched the keys of an accordeon and played the instrument, while the medium's hands were visible meantime, and even held at times by persons seated near him.

"The hands and fingers have always appeared solid and like those of any living person; at times, however, they appeared nebular, condensations in the form of hands.

"These phenomena were not visible to the same extent to all the persons present. For example, one person would see a flower or other small object; another person would see a small cloud of luminosity fly over the flower; another, still, would notice a nebulous hand; while others, again, would simply see the movement of the flower.

"I have seen, on several occasions, an object move with the appearance of a luminous cloud and perfectly condense into the form of a hand; under such circumstances the hand is visible to all persons present.

"It is not always a simple form, for often the hand perfectly resembles that of a living person, and has every element of grace; the fingers move; the flesh presents a human appearance, the same as though that of a living person; at the wrist or arm this form may become nebulous, and end in a luminous cloud of vapor.

"To the touch the hand appears cold, icy as in death at times; while on other occasions it feels warm and living, clasping my hand like that of an old friend would.

"I have retained one of these hands in mine, *firmly resolved not to let it escape*; it made no resistance nor effort to disengage itself, but appeared to gradually resolve itself into vapor." (*Crookes*).

I have heard many persons affirm that they perceived hands that touched them in *full light*. I never had this experience, but I can testify that during eight or ten sittings I and five or six persons who assisted me felt these hands perfectly; and among these hands were those belonging to a small child, and *certainly* no small child was in the house; these baby hands were soothing and caressing. Our medium was still Madam L. B., who, during the *seance*, was held down tightly on a sofa by Madam P., whose scrupulous attention may be relied on where *science* is at stake, for all our experimentations of this sort were in the dark. Several times the small baby hands were put in my sleeve, and seemed to take pleasure in pulling off my cuffs and taking them to other persons in the room. My eyeglass was also taken by the infantile fingers and carried to one of the circle.[87]

CLASS X.—*Direct writing.*

This is the expression we employ to designate a writing not produced by any person present, and Mr. Crookes gives the following description of this phenomenon:

"I have often received words and messages written on paper (on which I had made private marks) under the most severe conditions of control; and I have heard, in the dark, the noise of the pencil moving across the paper. The precautions previously taken by me were so strict that my mind is perfectly convinced, as if the characters of the writing were formed under my own eyes.

"But, as space will not permit me to enter into complete details, I shall simply choose two cases in which my eyes as well as my ears were witnesses of the operation.

"The first case I shall cite took place, it is true, in *dark seance*, but the result was none the less satisfactory.

"I was seated near the medium, Miss Fox, and there were only two persons present, my wife and a relative of ours; I held both hands of the medium in one of mine, while her feet were on top of my own. There was paper before us on the table and my hand held the pencil.

"A luminous hand descended from above, and, after hovering near me for a few seconds, took the pencil from my hand, writing rapidly on the paper, threw the pencil over our heads and gradually faded in obscurity.

"The second case may be considered and registered as a discovery. A good discovery is often more convincing than the most successful experiment.

"This occurred in the light of my own room, in the presence of Mr. Home and a few friends. Different circumstances, unnecessary to enumerate here, had shown that evening that *the psychic power was very strong*. I expressed the desire of witnessing the production of a real written message, similar to that I had one of my friends mention a short time before. At the instant this wish was uttered an alphabetical communication was given which read, '*We will try.*'

"A pencil and some sheets of paper were placed on the center of the table. Soon *the pencil stood on its point and advanced*, by jerks, then fell over. It raised itself again and fell over; it tried a third time but with no better result.

"After three fruitless attempts, a small piece of wood which laid near on the table slid towards the pencil and raised itself some inches above the table. The pencil now raised itself anew, supporting itself against the wood, and the two made an effort to write on the paper; this did not succeed and a new trial was made. On the third attempt the wooden lath abandoned its efforts and fell back to its old position on the table; the pencil remained in the position where it fell on the paper, and an alphabetical message said to us, "*We have tried to do what you have asked, but our power is exhausted.*" (Crookes.)

In India, the Fakirs easily obtain direct writing; they spread fine sand on a table or other smooth surface and place on this sand a small pointed stick made of wood. At a given moment this stick rises and traces characters on the sand, which are responses to questions put by the lookers on.[88]

In the experiments made with our friend Dr. Puel, we obtained writing on over twenty slates. A bit of chalk was placed on a new slate and this slate was placed on a table at some distance from the medium, Madam L. B., the experiments being made with all the cautions possible. A previous examination of both surfaces of the slate put away all doubts as to any fraud in that respect. I, meantime, held the hands of Madame L. B., the medium, who was always in a hypnotic condition during such experiments, at which several persons usually assisted—persons who were known to be capable of observing and recording facts with coolness and deliberation.

All these communications have a signature, and many of them date 1900 as the epoch when *modern spiritualism* shall be scientifically recognized by the world.

Dr. Gibier, who made interesting experiments with Mr. Slade, like us, obtained spontaneous writing on many slates, of which he gives reproductions in his remarkable work, *a book that he had the courage to write and to which his celebrated name is affixed.*[89]

We do not find in any Middle Age documents such spontaneously written communications; at least Demonographers do not mention them in their writings, for if they had it would have been a most striking proof of the analogy of magic with modern spiritualism and Indian Fakirism, which serves as an intermediary in the history of Occultism.

CLASS XI.—*Forms and figures of phantoms.*

"These phenomena are rarely ever witnessed. The conditions required for their appearance seeming so delicate, and so little prevents their production, that it is only on very few occasions that I have witnessed satisfactory results. I will cite two cases:

"At twilight, in a *seance* by Mr. Home, given at a private house, the blinds of a window, back of the medium about eight feet, were seen to move, then all the persons sitting near the window perceived a shadowy form that grew darker and then semi-transparent, like that of a man trying the shutters with his hand. While we gazed at this object in the twilight it evanesced and the window shutters ceased to move.

"The following example is still more striking. As in the preceding case Mr. Home was the medium. A phantom form came from the corner of the room, took an accordeon in its hand, and glided around the room playing the instrument beautifully. This phantom was visible to all those present for the space of several minutes, Mr. Home being perfectly visible at the same time. Then this shade approached a lady in the room, when the frightened woman uttered a scream and the phantom vanished." (*Crookes.*)

We regret that space will not permit our giving the experiments made on Miss Cook and Katie King, spectres which became so tangible that they were photographed.

This History given by Crookes regarding spiritual photography is well nigh incredible, but Dr. Crookes has remarked concerning doubters and his personal experiments, "*I do not say that it is possible, I say that it is.*"

These apparitions of forms and figures of phantoms were more common to the Middle Ages than at the present day, if we are to believe the numerous cases cited by Pierre Le Loyer.[90]

This celebrated author in fact, will not admit that there is any doubt on this subject; a matter he has thoroughly studied, for he says in this preface of his work—*"Aussi est traicte des extases et rauissements: de l'essence, nature et origine des Ames, et de leur estat apres le deces de leurs corps; plus des Magiciens et Sorciers, de leur communication avec les malins esprits; ensemble des remedes pour se preseruer des illusions et impostures diaboliques."*

In analyzing passages from this curious document, we will immediately see the correlation that exists between what was called in other times sorcery or magic, and spiritualism. In speaking of these spectres which form in the air, and under our eyes, Pierre Le Loyer writes: "We know them by the coldness of their touch and their bodies, which are soft, their hands receding from ours like soft cotton when pressed, or a snow-ball squeezed in a child's hand. They tarry no longer than it pleases them, returning again into their element."

Further along, Le Loyer adds: "A bad spirit questioned by a sorcerer why his body was not warm, responded that it was not in his power to give it heat."

But, meantime, he attributed these apparitions to evil spirits and demons; finally, our author seeks to explain "what is this body seen and touched of these demons, so to speak, of the air, water and earth?"

"These devils appear indifferently to all persons; they themselves affect the society of certain, individuals some much more than others."

"To these sorcerers and witches (*mediums*), they ordinarily show themselves in a visible form, and will come to those who call them."

"As to persons subject to these sort of things, they are usually those young and tender of age, cold and imperfectly organized beings; by such we can speak with power; old men and eunuchs, and withal melancholy persons."

"All those these devils dominate over, are estranged from their natural, beings, and not infrequently become maniacs."

Our author in his chapter on the essence of souls, affirms, that "that the ancient oracles *were only the Oracles of the souls of men,*" and to be specific, he gives a long list of names. He remarks, "there were in Greece, temples known to be psychomantic, and in such places were received responses from the souls of different men. It was for this reason too, that the souls for the same reason watched over the places where the bodies of generous and noble barons had been burned."

Further along Le Loyer mentions the origin of the *power that the spirits possess of manifesting themselves to us*, but our author *disagrees with the modern theories that makes them derive their power from the medium*, for he remarks that the spirits can act *"through their own powers,"* and are governed only by their own intelligence. "They are not off so far," adds he, "and the distance between us and the spirits is so slight that we may easily communicate;" however, he says, meantime: "They are commanded by God and conform to his will."

Finally, he considers man as an inferior being to the spirits of the dead—in fact, he states: "The soul appears to derive nothing from another, and, as an invisible spirit, it acts with us as a passive agent, being too proud to control that which is inferior; and I deny," says he, "that the true souls of the dead obey either charms or magical words."

Of the future of the soul after death he remarks to one of his opponents, whose opinions he refuted, that *"this soul, whatever it may be, in a state of health or not purged, comes by degrees and not at one bound into the full fruition and happiness of God;"* and these degrees, according to Le Loyer, are like prisons where the penalties for misdeeds done in the flesh are to be satisfied. He admits, however, that some spirits make more rapid progress than others. These, to his mind, are the judgments of God after death, and the fire mentioned in Scriptures. Such is the manner in which he explains away the ideas of the images of Paradise and Hell, the promises to the virtuous and the wicked. He cites (*apropos* of manifestations before courts of justice) houses "where spirits have appeared and made all manner of noises, that disturbed the tenants at night." He speaks of Daniel and Nicholas Macquereau, who rented a house for a term of years. "They had been living there but a short time when they heard the noises and hubbub made by invisible spirits, who allowed them neither sleep nor repose." The court cancelled the lease, thus *admitting that there were places haunted by spirits."*[91]

CLASS XII.—*Particular examples which seem to indicate the intervention of a superior intelligence.*

"It has already been demonstrated that these phenomena are governed by an Intelligence; an important question is to know what is the source of this Intelligence.

"Is this the Intelligence of the *medium* or some one else present in the room? Or is this Intelligence exterior? I do not wish to commit myself on this point at present in a positive manner. I will say that I have observed several circumstances which appeared to demonstrate that the will and the intelligence of the medium have a great influence on the phenomena. I have likewise observed others which seemed to prove in a conclusive manner the intervention of an intelligence entirely independent of all persons found in the room where the *seance* was given.

"Space will not permit me to give here all the arguments that might serve to prove these propositions, but I will briefly mention one or two circumstances chosen from among a number of others. I have several times seen phenomena take place simultaneously, some of them being unknown to the medium. I have seen Miss Fox write automatically a message for a person present, while a message for another person was given alphabetically by means of *raps*, and during all the time of these manifestations she conversed on a subject entirely different from the two others.

"The following case is, perhaps, still more astonishing. During a *seance* with Mr. Home, a small wooden lath, that I have previously mentioned, came across the table to me, in full light, and gave me a message by striking lightly on my hand; I repeated the alphabet and the lath struck me at the proper letters; the other end of this wooden stick was some distance off from the hands of Mr. Home.

"The blows were so distinct and clear, the wooden lath was so evidently under the invisible power that governed its movements, that I said: 'Can the intelligence that governs the movements of this lath change the character of the movement and give me a telegraphic message by means of the Morse alphabet, by blows struck on my hand?'

"I had every reason for thinking that the Morse alphabet was entirely unknown to all the other persons present, and I knew it only imperfectly myself.

"Immediately after I had said this the character of the raps changed and the message was continued in the manner I demanded. The letters were given too rapidly for me to catch but a word now and then, consequently I lost the message; but I had heard sufficient to convince me that there was a good Morse operator at the other extremity of the line, no matter what place it might be in.

"Another example: A lady wrote automatically by the aid of Planchette. I sought to discover the means to prove what she wrote was not due to *unconscious cerebration*. Planchette, as it always does, affirmed that, although the movements were made by the hands and arms of the operator, there was an intelligence coming from an invisible being, who played on her brain like an instrument of music and thus put her muscles in motion.

"I then remarked to this Intelligence, 'Can you see what is contained in this chamber?' And Planchette answered, 'Yes.' 'Can you read this journal?' said I, placing my finger on a copy of the *London Times* that happened to be back of me on a table, but which I could not see. 'Yes' responded Planchette. 'Very well,' said I, 'write the word now covered by my finger.' Planchette commenced to move and the word 'however' was slowly written. I turned around and saw that the word 'however' was covered by the end of my finger. I had not looked at the paper when I attempted this experiment, and it was impossible for the lady, had she tried, to see any word in the journal, as she was seated at a table and the *London Times* lay on a table back of me with my body interposed." (*Crookes.*)

In the experiments in typtology at which I have assisted, to all the demands addressed to *psychic force* the responses have always presented a particular character independent of that of the assistants.[92]

I have sometimes tried to concentrate my will upon the answer awaited, and have always failed in my attempts at mental pressure.

1 have likewise determined that these answers cannot be dictated by the mind of the medium, whose scientific and literary knowledge were not always equal to the message received. This observation coincides with the facts observed among pretended Demonomaniacs, who had in their attacks the gift of language, responding in Latin to the exorcists, making entire discourses in this language, of which they knew not the first elements.

Under the name of *phenomena of ecstasy*, Dr. Gibier described, after his experiments with the medium Slade, his displacement by a stronger spirit to that of his usual control. Says Gibier, the phenomena produced from thence were "a certain discoloration of the medium's face, which became red, a sort of grin contracting the muscles of the visage, the eyes were convulsed upwards, and after some nystagmatic movements of the ball of the eye the eyelids closed tightly, gritting of the medium's teeth was heard, and a convulsive sign, indicating the commencement of his *possession* by a strange spirit. After this short phase, which was painful to behold, the medium's face fell into a smile and the voice, as well as the attitude, was completely modified to that of a different person. Slade thus transformed to his regular control, saluted all our party most graciously."

Among the experiments made by Dr. Gibier to control this condition of *incarnation* (the English call it *trance*), we might cite that of a comparison of the dynamometric force of the medium in his natural condition and the *trance* state. In the first case, by reason of two previous attacks of hemiplegia, Slade's muscular force gave 27 kilos to the right and 35 kilos to the left. In the second state there were 63 kilos to the right and 50 kilos to the left. Meantime, Dr. Gibier, no more than ourselves, deems it proper to consider the trance state other than a hypothesis, "a foreign element, introduced in the scene, and like it present in the experiences of suggestion and catalepsy."

If we cannot give a scientific explanation of these phenomena, it is our duty to examine them as others and retrace their history, especially seeking those points of coincidence with the proofs furnished by the history of demonomania and diabolic possession of the Middle Ages; for we are convinced that these phenomena were dominated by the same unknown force, interpreted differently by reason of the philosophic and religious ideas of the epoch at which they were studied.

CLASS XIII.—*Varied cases of a complex character.*

Under this title Mr. Crookes cites facts that cannot be classed otherwise by reason of their complex character. As an example, he reports two cases: one being an experiment in typtology between himself, Miss Fox, and another lady. He proved that a bell that belonged in his business office was brought to the table, as a proof announced by the intellectual force, that communicated with him, *of its strength.* The chamber in which this was done was separated from the office by a door which he previously securely locked with a key, and he was absolutely positive that the bell in question was in his office.

"The second case I desire to report," says Mr. Crookes, "took place one Saturday night under a full glare of light, Mr. Home and my family being the only persons present.

"My wife and I, having passed the day in the country, had brought home flowers with us that I had gathered; on arriving at home we had given them to a servant to put in water. Mr. Home came shortly after and we went into the dining room. At the instant we seated ourselves, the domestic brought the flowers, arranged in a vase; I placed them in the center of the table, which was not covered by a cloth. It was the first time Mr. Home had seen these flowers.

"Immediately a message came, given by the rap alphabet, which said, 'It is impossible for matter to pass through matter, but we will show you that we can do it.' We waited in silence, and soon a luminous apparition was seen floating over the bouquet of flowers, and then, in full view of all my family at the table, a branch of China grass, fifteen inches in length, which ornamented the middle of the bouquet, slowly rose from the bunch of flowers, descended from the vase and moved across the table, and my wife saw a hand stretched out from under the table and seize the flower; at the same moment she was struck three times on the left shoulder and the noise made by the slaps was so loud we all heard it; then the luminous hand dropped the China grass to the floor and disappeared. Only two persons of my family saw the hand, but every one at the table noticed the different movements of the plant stalk, as I have before described them.

"During the time that this phenomena lasted we all saw Mr. Home's hands on the table, where they rested motionless, and they were at least eighteen inches from where the plant stalk disappeared.

"It was a dining-room table that opened in folds, it did not lengthen," etc.

As a contribution to the facts mentioned in this class, I may report the famous experiments with the bracelet made by Dr. Puel—experiments that I have witnessed a dozen times at least—as well as numerous other persons. A bracelet made of brass, without opening or solder, cut by a machine out of a solid piece of metal, was placed on the forearm of Madame L. B. The lady's hands rested flat on the table, or were held in the hands of those experimenting. At a given moment, often in the middle of a conversation, Madame L. B. uttered a piercing cry and at the same instant the bracelet would fall on the floor, or on some piece of furniture, with great force. Several times, under the same circumstances,—that is to say, when the lady's hands were firmly pressed down on the table by those experimenting,—I have seen the bracelet *pass from one arm to the other.*

So, in opposition to all laws of physics, it appears that matter can pass through matter; I affirm the reality of this, and others, who are no more victims to hallucination than I, can also testify to the truth of this statement. And no matter what may be the consequences to my professional reputation, and utterly without regard for anything that may be said by critics, I boldly maintain, as if under oath, that my senses lead me to this imposed conviction. Besides, I am far from being alone in believing what I have seen, whether or no it be *"in harmony with our acquired knowledge;"* to the names of French, English and German *savants* I have cited, there are experimenters in all countries who have the courage to believe the evidence offered by their own senses, as witness that celebrated English geologist, who, after ten years of investigation with the phenomena under control, *declared spiritualism to be true,* drawing from his experiments the following conclusions: *"Who shall determine the limits of the possible, limits that science and observation accumulate each day? Let us examine, let us doubt, but not be so daring as to deny the possibility of such occurrences"* (Barkas).

If now we have established the balance-sheet of facts attributed to the Demonomania of the Middle Ages, and compared them to the experiences of experimental psychology, we are not only led to recognize a striking analogy between them, but also to interpret them by the hypothesis of an intelligent force of an intensity proportionate to certain nervous pathological conditions. It is necessary to remember, in fact, that, according to the Ritual of the Roman Catholic Church, the phenomena necessary to recognize *possession* among Demonomaniacs were:

1. The faculty of knowing thoughts, even though they are not expressed.

2. Intelligence in unknown languages.

3. The faculty of speaking foreign tongues which are unknown to the party speaking them.

4. A knowledge of future events.

5. A knowledge of what is transpiring in far-off places.

6. Development of superior psychal force.

7. Suspension of persons or bodies in the air for a considerable space of time.

No less interesting is it than to compare these phenomena to those observed by the thirty-three members of the commission appointed by the "Dialectic Society of London." The following was this committee's report, after eighteen months' investigation:

1. Noises of varied nature, apparently arising from the furniture, floor or walls of the room, accompanied by vibrations which are often perceptible to the touch, are present without being produced by muscular action or any mechanical means whatever.

2. Movements of heavy bodies occur without the aid of mechanical apparatus of any sort, and without equivalent development of muscular force on the part of persons present, and even frequently without contact or connection with any one.

3. These noises and movements are produced often at the moment wished for and in the manner demanded by persons present, and, by means of a simple code of sounds, respond to questions and write coherent communications.

4. The response and communications obtained are, for the most part, hackneyed and commonplace, but sometimes they give facts and information only known to one person in the room.

5. The circumstances under which the phenomena are present vary, the most striking feature being that the presence of certain persons seems necessary to their production, and that the presence of some people serves as a check; but this difference does not seem to depend on the belief or the unbelief of those present as to the nature of the phenomena.

The testimony, oral and written, received by the commission affirmed the reality of phenomena much more extraordinary still, such as heavy bodies rising in the air (men in certain cases floated through the atmosphere) and remaining in suspension without tangible support; apparitions of hands and forms belonging to no human beings, but seemingly alive, judging by their aspect and motions.

This report was signed by *savants* of the first order, as sceptical before commencing their investigations as the most positive Materialists of our academies of science. Let us cite, among the celebrated names of men known throughout the world for their learning and scientific veracity, those of the great naturalist and *collaborateur* of Darwin, Russell Wallace, Professor A. Morgan, President of the Mathematical Society of London and Secretary of the Royal Astronomical Society; F. Varley, Chief Engineer of the Trans-Atlantic Telegraph Company and member of the Royal Society of London.

Mr. Morgan does not fear to add to the report the following lines: "I am perfectly convinced, from what I have seen and heard, in a manner that renders doubt impossible, that *Spiritualists*, without doubt, are upon a track that will lead to the advancement of the psychal sciences; their opponents are those who seek to trammel all progress."

Mr. Varley writes to the celebrated Professor Tyndall: "I am obliged to investigate the nature of the force that produces these phenomena, but, up to the present time, I have been unable to discover anything save the source from which this *psychic force* emanates, *i.e.*, from the vital systems of the mediums. I am only studying, however, a thing that has been the object of investigation for two thousand years; brave men, whose minds are elevated above the narrow prejudices of our century, seem to have sounded the depths of the subject in question," etc.

This opinion of the learned English physicist proves, once more, that we are right in connecting Demonomania to the magic of antiquity and to modern spiritualism. One must be perfectly blind or of poor judgment not to see the connecting links that unite these various phenomena. And if our men of science dare no longer say that these facts are worthy of credit, although refusing to investigate the same, it is because they lack courage, it is because they dare not brave the criticism of pretended strong-minded men and the jests of the ignorant. If the *vulgum pecus*, the amorphous matter that stuffs the superior element of society, contest the value of the works of Crookes, Wallace, Morgan, Varley, Gibier, Zoellner, Mapes, Hare, Oxon, Sexton, and others, they can only be included in the same class of people who ridiculed Galileo, Harvey, Jenner, Franklin, Young, Davy, Jussieu, Papin, Stephenson, and Galvani, with all the authors of great discoveries and scientific truths, who have invariably been combatted by the pseudo-scientific and half-fledged goslings whose names adorn our so-called colleges and other mutual admiration societies.[93]

Why, then, longer refuse to study *a force* recognized by some of the most eminent men among modern civilized nations and by the modest pioneers who first studied these phenomena in France? If the number of experimenters named be not sufficient to convince sceptics, let them enter into a full study of present-day psychology, and find a host of the greatest modern neurologists.

Nine years of study has led Mr. Oxon, Professor at the University of Oxford, to formulate the following propositions on *Psychic Force*, which corroborate the results obtained by his colleagues in England, Germany, and America, and which still constitute another proof of the identity of the phenomena:

"1. A force exists which acts by means of a special type of human organization, a force that we call *psychic force*.

"2. It is demonstrated that this force is, in certain cases, governed by an intelligence.

"3. It is proved that this intelligence is often other than that of the person or persons through whose influence it acts.

"4. This Force, thus governed by an exterior intelligence, at times manifests its action, independent of other methods, by writing coherent phrases, without the intervention of any known mode of writing.

"5. The evidence of the existence of this force governed by an intelligence rests on

"(*a*) The evidence observed through the senses.

"(*b*) The fact that *the force* often uses a language unknown to the medium.

"(*c*) The fact that the subject matter treated is very frequently superior to the medium's knowledge or education.

"(*d*) The fact that it has been found impossible to produce the same results by fraud under the conditions in which these phenomena are obtained.

"(*e*) The fact that these special phenomena are not only produced in public and by paid mediums, but likewise in a family circle where no strangers are admitted."

Without writing to prejudice the question, I believe, in my turn, that I can solemnly affirm that this force has intimate connection with the soul, the mind or the ministerial part of our being, as it is called; that it acts on our ideas as well as on our physiological functions, and it is to my mind the destiny of humanity to investigate its essence and study its phenomena, its manifestations and all its sensible effects by all our senses and means of investigation.

It is high time that secular boasting of the materialistic scientists be checked, and that they should recognize the fact that force does not arise from matter alone but exists independent of it and primarily submits to its laws.

Starting, then, with the proposition that an unknown force exists, to whose influence we unconsciously submit, science should investigate this force, isolate, and control it, if it be in our power so to do.

Instead of opposing an ignorant skepticism to modern discoveries in *psychic force*, our learned Academicians should investigate the acquired facts for inspiration in future work, remembering that good thought of Laplace: "We are so far from knowing all the agents of Nature and their different modes of action, that it is not philosophical to deny the existence of phenomena simply because they cannot be explained in the actual condition of our present knowledge."[94]

Such are the conclusions I believe I have a right to draw from my historical studies on the Demonomania of the Middle Ages. Let me briefly recapitulate my personal views on the subject:

1. There exists a psychic force, intelligent, inherent to humanity, manifesting itself, under determined conditions, by various phenomena, with an intensity more or less great.

2. Certain human beings, known as mediums, who are very sensitive to the action of magnetism, facilitate the production of these phenomena, considered as supernatural in the actual state of our present scientific knowledge, and in apparent contradiction with all known physical and physiological laws.

3. In certain nervous conditions, natural or provoked, this Force can possess the human organism and bring about, temporarily, either a change in one's personality or an alteration in one's sensations and in the intellectual and moral faculties.

MEDICINE IN THE LITERATURE OF THE MIDDLE AGES.

All *savants* who have studied the literary and historical part of medicine fully recognize the powerful interest it offers, especially that medicine portrayed in the works of poets and dramatic authors of the Middle Ages. It is in the works of these writers, in fact, that we find the most exact appreciation of medical ideas of the epoch, because we can judge their morals, criticise their faults, account for their tendencies—all without bringing in medical science at any given moment, with its teachings, errors, and prejudices.

In all that concerns the Middle Ages, we shall find this first in the writings of philosophers, in certain dramatic works, known under the name of *Moralities*, because their purport was to demonstrate, under the form of an allegory, a precept of morality. The personages of such dramatic scenes always represent ideas, often abstract and usually fantastic,—The World, Justice, Good Company, Gourmands, Dinner, Banquet, Experience, Gout, Jaundice, Dropsy, and Apoplexy. A second class, errors and prejudices, are seldom wanting in some poetical works, in *comedies and farces*, *satirical* and *indecent* poems, that recall some of the early productions of the Latin Theatre. Eventually impressed with the Gallic spirit of levity, these short pieces, enjoyed by clerks and small tradesmen, contain cutting criticisms on the weaknesses of mankind, doctors in particular. These plays are considered the embryo of the French stage, which, later, has been immortalized by the most illustrious of our writers of comedy.

An unaffected gayety often breaks out in brilliant, sparkling dialogues in these frivolous farces, and assures the instant success of the play. The public laughed in high glee, without prudery, at the broad I insinuations and comical acts in such representations. So the writers of that period went into raptures when they chanced to make a hit with their satirical tirades, that amused the passing age. Sometimes the clergy were satirized as well as the doctor; even the Pope himself received the attention of the comedians, as witness the carnival of 1511. Even the avarice of Louis XII. was ridiculed. Comedy's procession represented Justice by its attorneys, shysters and police; but, above all, comedy delighted to burlesque the doctor, *Facultas saluberrema medicinæ parisiensis*, ridiculing them like the rest of the world, without the least respect for their robe or bonnet.

Pray, what do these jolly, railing spirits of the Middle Ages say of our medical ancestors of the good old times? Master Jehan Bouchet, for example, with his piece, *Traverseur des voyes perilleuses*, and Pierre Gringore under the pseudonym of *Mere Sotte*, and Nicholas Rousset and Coustellier, and Jacques Grevin and Pierre Blanchet, and all other members of that joyous group without care, without pretension, but not without talent. If professional honor was never really put on trial by these wits, the pedantic gravity of our medical forefathers, their formidable doctoral accoutrement, their consultations, sentences formulated in horrible and barbarous Latin, were all the objects of raillery and piquant epigrams. We shall find also, in other works we propose to analyze, the same false ideas of the public regarding the healing art as exists to-day; the same tendency to always lead one into error, and unjustly accuse the medical profession of all the accidents that happen to a patient—this, too, notwithstanding all ancient codes of hygiene and all the ages of experience.

When a physician prescribed, for example, in the case of one attacked by fever, the daily libations were stopped, and we always find the neighbors and boon companions of the sufferer enter the sick room for the purpose of criticizing the doctor's prescriptions and orders, and such persons excited the patient by their remarks on medical despotism. This has always been the case since doctors and patients were created, not only in the Middle Ages, but at all epochs. Olivier Basselin bears testimony to this fact in one of his charming *Vaux de Vire*[95] poetical compositions, roundelays and Bacchic songs, dating back to the sixteenth century; this sonnet is not long;[96] it relates to a drunkard to whom only barley water is given, and who recovers his health, according to the veracious poet, through a charitable friend, who breaks the doctor's orders and fills the patient up with wine. We have often read this poem with pleasure, and give a condensed extract:

One of my neighbors sick was lying,

Gasping with weak and feverish breath:

"Alas! they'll kill me," said he, sighing,

"Forbidding wine; and barley water's death.

"Alas! my thirst is great, annoying;

I'd like one drink before I die;

Neighbor, with you one glass enjoying;

Pray quickly to the vintner's hie.

"Dear friend, my wish don't be denying,

Always to me you've been a brother;

Now, for the wine in haste go flying,

We'll take one parting glass together.

"Since doctors made me quit a-drinking,

My flask I've left yon in my will.

These doctors, I can't help a-thinking,

Don't cure as often as they kill."

Thus spoke my neighbor, sick and weary.

Of wine he drank full bottles five;

The fever left him blithe and cheery;

He's still a-drinking, and *alive*.

The Bibliotheque of the French Theatre contains a great number of other dramatic compositions, as well as comedies and farces, in which doctors carry principal *roles*, it is true, but more often are introduced for the mere purpose of giving the author a chance for pleasantry at the expense of medicine; and these characters sometimes exceed the limit of license. Some of these works are gems of literary art. We may cite, for instance, the "Farce of the Doctor who Cures all Diseases," by Nicholas Rousset; the "Discours Facetieux" of Coustellier; "The true Physician, who Cures all Known Diseases;" and several besides, "La Medecine de Maistre Grimache," "Le Triomphe de treshaulte et tres puissante Dame Verolle," of Francois Juste; "Mary and the Doctor," "The Sweetheart of the Family Physician," as well as some farces by Tabarin—works dating back to the fifteenth, sixteenth and seventeenth centuries.

But we shall only take up the study of a few works that have a veritable literary medical interest, and shall confine ourselves to the study of the "Farces de Maitre Pathelin, du Munyer et de la Folie du Monde;" to the moralities of "A'aveugle et du Boiteux, de Folie et d'Amour;" to the comedies of "La Tresoriere et de Lucelle;" to the tragedy "De la Goutte," and to the book of "Gargantua et de Pantagruel." This will suffice to give an idea of medicine as portrayed in the literature of the Middle Ages.

THE FARCE OF MASTER PATHELIN.

The farce of Master Pathelin, whose author was Pierre Blanchet, is certainly the richest jewel in the crown of the old French Theatre; it was what inspired Moliere in several of his works. Represented for the first time in 1480, this celebrated farce is one of the most precious literary monuments for the study of Middle Age morality. It is a *chef d'œuvre* of spirit, malice, comedy, and *naivete*, in which medicine is found in every scene, either in the simulation of disease, with consultations, with drugs, and, most amusing of all, the eternal ingratitude of the sick.

All the educated world knows the subject of Master Pathelin: A lawyer without a case or client; a man living on his wits and expedients, making dupes and yet retaining a certain degree of professional correctness in his language and his artifices. Guillemette, his wife, is his worthy accomplice. It is she who reproaches him with not having more clients and his reputation of earlier days; of starving her to death by famine. It is she who excites him by ironically saying:

"Maintenant chascun vous appelle

Partout; avocat dessoubz l'orme,

Nos robes sont plus qu'estamine

Reses."

And Pathelin responds that he cannot get their clothing out of pawn without redeeming or stealing it—both things out of the question, as he has no money and will not commit a crime. It is then that the worthy couple hit on the credit system to renew their wardrobe. It is for this purpose he goes to a draper's to purchase cloth to make new clothes. On entering the shop he uses the salutation of the period, "God be with you," and politely inquires after the shopkeeper's health, which to him is very dear. Then he asks after his father's health, telling him he resembles his sire like an old picture. Finally, he takes sixteen yards of fine cloth, and, telling the draper to call at his house in the evening for his money and to eat, as Master Pathelin expresses it, "a Rouen goose roasted," having invited the astonished tradesman to dine with him, the lawyer walks out with the cloth without paying. Arriving home he relates his adventure to the delighted Guillemette, who is overpowered with bewilderment, however, when she learns that the draper is invited to a roast goose supper. At first it is suggested that they borrow a tailor's goose, but fear that the draper will not appreciate the joke and demand his money legally induces the worthy couple to adopt a strategem. It is very simple: Master Pathelin is to feign insanity, or rather that maniacal form of excitation so frequently employed even at the present day by those who seek to avoid the consequences of crimes—an excitation principally characterized by uncontrollable loquacity, mobility of ideas, incoherence, and pretended illusions.

These scenes of simulation are extremely curious and interesting. As soon as the draper enters the wife warns him not to make a noise in the house:

"He's lying in bed. Don't speak!

Poor martyr! he's been sick a week.

But the draper refuses to accept the explanation. It cannot be a week, he says, for

"'Tis only this afternoon, you see,

Your husband bought cloth from me."

Then the voice of the attorney is heard in the next room shouting to his wife:

"Guillemette? Un peu d'eue rose!

Haussez moy, serrez-moy derriere!

Trut! a qui parlay. Je? L'esguiere?

A boire? Frottez moy la plante."

Rose water in that century was employed to reanimate the strength of sick people. Among apothecaries it was called *aqua cordialis temperata*. Rose water was prescribed in the following cases: "*In mortis subitis et malignis, ubicunque magnus est virium lapsus præscribitur; quemadmodum etiam prodest a morbo convalescentibus, ad vires instaurandas.*"

Pathelin simulates hallucinations of sight, and uses all manner of words employed by magicians in their conjurations; he asks the draper and Guillemette to put a charm around his neck such as are used to frighten away demons. He then, in his ravings, abuses the doctors for their malpractice and not understanding the quality of his urine.([197]) Notwithstanding all this the draper is not convinced and demands his money. We all know what importance was attributed to the examination of the urine in olden times, long before any search was made for albumen, sugar, or other morbid principles that it might contain. Charlatans especially exploited in this field of medicine, practicing it illegally in the country under the name of *water jugglers* or *water judges*. Such men still practice in Normandy and certain northern provinces of France.

The intestinal functions had also more or less importance in the eyes of the public, and the physician was not always consulted as when to give physic. People sent to an apothecary and ordered a clyster with cassia and other ingredients, according to the following formula of the pharmacopœia: "*Cassia Pro Clysteribus. Est eadem pulpa cassiæ cum decocto herbarum aperitirarum extracta et saccharo Thomæo condita. Oportet autem illas herbas adhibere recentes, parumque decoquere, alias viribus aperitivis omnio privantur; siccæ autem per se carent virtute illa aperitiva.*"

In the "Revue Historique" of Angers we find a document bearing on the private life of Cardinal Richelieu; it has for its title: "Things furnished for the person of His Most Eminent Highness, the Cardinal Duke Richelieu during the year 1635, by Perdreau, apothecary to his Excellency." During the one year the Cardinal had used seventy-five clysters and twenty-seven cassia boluses, without counting other laxative medicines and bottles of tisane, his purgative bill amounting to 1401 livres and 14 sous. It is evident that Richelieu was a badly constipated Cardinal.

It was a fine period for apothecaries, and we might add that Moliere did them considerable harm.

Let us return to Master Pathelin. He was allowed a short breathing spell for Guillemette, fought off the obdurate creditor by making him leave the room a few moments while her husband used the bedpan.

But this respite is of short duration; the draper soon returns to demand his cloth back or his money, although the wife declares her husband "is dying in frenzy." Then commences another scene of maniacal simulation in this wonderful psychological play. In his pretended delirium, Pathelin indulges in Limousin *patois*, Flemish, Lower Breton; his words grow unintelligible and incoherent in order to convince the draper of his insanity.

"Mere de Diou, la coronade,

Par fie, y m'en voul anar,

Or renague biou, outre mar,

Ventre de Diou, zen diet gigone,

Castuy carrible, et res ne donne."

Let us pass from a wild Flemish harangue, that possesses but little interest even to those understanding the dialects.

The psychic symptoms, which dominate in the simulated delirium of Master Pathelin, are especially incoherent in language with mobility of ideas. The author of this fine comedy had evidently observed the progressive instability of thought among certain maniacs, the impossibility of fixing their attention, the too rapid succession of ideas without order; in fact, that absolute incoördination, a kind of cerebral automatism, which is the announcement of the breaking-down of intellectual faculties and the prelude of absolute dementia. In his ravings, Pathelin descants on the *Mal de Saint Garbot*, or, more properly speaking, Garbold; this was dysentery, although such a scholar as Genin translates it as meaning hemorrhoids. Saint Garbold who was Bishop of Bayeux in the seventh century, was driven out from his episcopal chair by his diocesans, and, in order to be avenged, sent them dysentery.

We may remark, in this connection, that during the Middle Ages many maladies were called after the Saints, whose aid they invoked in given diseases; *Saint Ladre* or *Lazare*, for leprosy; *Saint Roch*, for the plague; *Saint Quentin*, for dropsy; *Saint Leu*, *Saint Loupt*, *Saint Mathelin*, *Saint Jehan*, *Saint Nazaire*, *Saint Victor*, for epilepsy, fever, deafness, madness, etc.

The *mal Saint Andreux*, *mal Saint Antoine*, *mal Saint Firmin*, *mal Saint Genevieve*, *mal Saint Germain*, *mal Saint Messaut*, *mal Saint Verain*, designated erysipelas, scurvy, etc. Drunkenness was called the *mal Saint Martin*.

Syphilis naturally had its patron Saint; in fact, it was known as *mal Saint homme Job*, *Saint Merais*, *Saint Laurant*, *mal Saint Eupheme*, etc. In fact, all diseases had as an attachment the name of one or more Saints, at whose shrine the afflicted might implore aid.

But to return to Master Pathelin: After numerous tirades he finishes by acknowledging his deceit to the draper. This is an epitome of the farce of Master Pierre Pathelin, a medical study that had an immense run in the fifteenth century and remains a valuable document regarding French morality in the Middle Ages, as interesting to the student of psychology as to the Theatre. Some years after this (1490) the sequel to Master Pathelin appeared, called the "Last Will of Pathelin," which is also full of strange medical conceits appertaining to the age in which it was written. In this piece, Pathelin, after years of fraud and deceit, really becomes ill and sends for the lawyer and priest, abandoning the doctor to a certain extent. In his will he leaves all his ailments to different religious orders and charitable institutions, as, for instance, one *item* of his will reads as follows:

"Au quatre convens aussi,

Cordeliers, Carmes, Augustins,

Jacobins, soient ors, on Soient ens,

Je leur laisse tous bons lopins,

A tous chopineurs et y vrongnes,

Notre vueil que je leur laisse

Toutes goutes, crampes et rongnes,

Au poing, au coste, a la fesse," etc.

But enough of Master Pathelin. Let us now turn to the consideration of another curious farce.

LA FARCE DE MUNYER.

This farce, whose author was Andre de la Vigne, dates back, like preceding one, to the fourteenth century. The miller of the Middle Ages, the ancestor of our present Jack-pudding (French slang for miller), was in antique times the most rascally and cheating type of trader, from whence the old Gascon proverb, "One always finds a thief in a miller's skin."

In this farce we see the miller "lying in bed as though sick," uttering long groans and sighing over the pains he professes to endure—groans, however, to which his wife appears insensible. He commences thus:

"Now am I in sore distress,

My sickness hard to cure,

My sore discomfort is not less.

Heart-ache I can't endure."

To this his wife responds indifferently, although the miller persists in asking for a bottle of good wine, saying that his "reins and belly need the supreme consolation of the bottle." The wife obstinately refuses her husband the wine, remarking that he cannot "repair his stomach by filling the belly;" but, instead, she sends for the priest, who is, moreover, her lover, and carries on a flirtation with the holy man in the presence of her husband, for the purpose of making the invalid rise from his sick-bed; but, thinking his end near, the miller demands that he shall be permitted to die in the faith, or "*mourir catholiquement.*" He confesses to the priest, avowing all his thefts, his frauds, his falsification and *amours*, and is prepared to render his soul.

But the miller has absorbed some of the popular ideas of his day, professed by certain philosophers of the time; he believes that, at the moment of death, the soul of man escapes by his anus, and warns the priest to absolve him from his sins, saying:

"Mon ventre trop se determine.

Helas! Je ne scay que je face;

Ostez vous!"

The priest answers:

"Ha! sauf vostre grace!"

Then the miller remarks:

"Ostez vous, car je me conchye."

The wife and the priest pull the sick man to the edge of the bed and place him in such a position that, if the doctrine of soul departure by the anus be true, they may witness the miller's final performance. The phenomenon of rectal flatulence is now observed, when suddenly to the consternation of the wife and priest, a demon appears, and placing a sack over the dying miller's anus catches the rectal gas and flies off in sulphurous vapor. In the next act we see the Devil appear before his patron Lucifer bearing the sack supposed to contain the damned soul of the miller received in the aforesaid sack at the moment it escaped from the anus. The devil is commanded by Lucifer to empty the sack at the feet of Proserpine who is busily engaged in cooking in Hell's kitchen, but in place of the miller's soul they only find *spoiled bran*; the rascal has cheated even in death.

It seems strange that earlier comedy writers all showed a tendency to make their principle scenes pathological burlesques. Thus in many plays the heroes and heroines were attacked by colic in order to excite the laughter of the audience, when the buffoon would imitate by signs the act of defecation. This peculiar French gayety and lack of prudery is fully evidenced in the comic effects of Pourceaugnac with the detersive, insinuative and carminative clysters of Moliere.

This farce, had in former days, an immense success, and is still occasionally played, being considered a *chef d'œuvre* of malice and humor by our best critics and most distinguished authors. In France the audience always laugh when a thief while plundering is suddenly taken with pains in his bowels and diarrhœa, while a rectal syringe flourished aloft as a weapon of defense will bring down the gallery in a storm of applause.

L'AVEUGLE ET LE BOITEUX

Is another play in which medicine acts a part, by the same author of the preceding farce; the plot is as follows: A blind man and a lame man implore public charity on a deserted road; the blind man deplores his fate as never having seen the light, and the lame man bitterly bemoans not being able to walk but a few steps at one time, on account of the gout which has rendered him paraplegic. These two make a mutual avowal of their infirmities and agree to form a copartnership for mutual assistance; the lame man climbs on the blind man's shoulders and they start out the road in search of charitable persons who may aid them with alms. On going some little distance the beggars hear a noise; this is made by a procession of monks going on a pilgrimage to the tomb of Saint Martin. "What do they say?" asks the blind man; to which the lame man responds:

They tell of things curious and quaint,

Of miracles, wonderous, if true,

Performed by a newly made saint,

For whose aid each monk goes to sue;

This Saint cures all ills he can find,

Even fits, ulcers, fevers and gout;

He *healeth the halt* and the blind

In a manner that's past finding out.

We all know the eternal popular faith and belief in the ability of the Saints to cure every malady that flesh is heir to. However, in the present instance, it seems that one of the requirements necessary to be healed was a perfect spirit of resignation to all ills on the part of the sufferer—*now this is the case of our two mendicants*, who now become alarmed at the idea that they may be cured and thus deprived of a method of earning their daily bread, *i.e.*, by beggary, so they undertake a number of subterfuges to escape the pious pilgrimage, which gives rise to many amusing adventures and situations, which might be well utilized by some modern playwriter. In the end the two mendicants escape from going with the pilgrim monks to visit the Saint's shrine, as the blind man detests the light and the lame man is too lazy to walk, in fact both are admirably suited with their afflictions. It is during one of these scenes that the lame man relates to the blind man the best methods for deceiving the public by simulating maladies, and making a regular profession of begging. He discloses all the secrets of those who in the Middle Ages sought public commiseration to earn alms; he remarks:

"Puisque de tout je suis reffait,

Maulgre mes deus et mon visage,

Tant feray, que seray deffaict,

Encore ung coup de mon corsaige,

Car je vous dis bien que encor scay—je"

"La grant pratique et aussi l'art,

Par onguement et par herbaige,

Combien que soye miste et gaillart,

Que huy on dira que ma jambe art

Du cruel mal de Sainct Anthoyne," etc.

In this lengthy poem, too long to transcribe from the French, the lame mendicant gives a list of herbs, through means of which various diseases may be simulated, especially those maladies of the skin that are repulsive to the majority of mankind; thus he describes the itch produced by certain varieties of the *clematis* and the appearance of leprosy induced by the use of an ointment of which *veronica* formed the basis. He also describes how to produce the disease of *Saint Fiacre*, an affection characterized by warts and ulcers around the anus. It is useless to add there is nothing new under the sun. Let us now turn our attention to another play, *i.e.*;

LUNACY AND LOVE.

This is a play with six characters, written in 1556, by Louise Labe, sometimes called the *Belle Cordiere*.

Love, at all periods of time, has served as an inexhaustible subject of analysis and observation, not only to poets and novelists, but also to moralists, and especially physicians. Psychologists have always considered love, when excessive, as an evidence of insanity. Esquirol says that "love has lost its empire in France, indifference having captivated the hearts of our people, who, given over to amorous passions, having neither purity nor exhaltation, engender attacks of erotic lunacy." This learned alienist has also discovered that out of 323 cases of insanity among the poor, love figured as a cause in forty-six cases; and out of 167 cases among the rich, twenty-five persons went insane on account of love. These close relations between "Lunacy and Love," admitted since mankind *entered into society*, have served as a text for the Middle Ages, as is witnessed by the title of the play we have mentioned; a work the more curious, for reason of its *finesse*, notwithstanding the jests employed by its author as the following analysis will witness.

Love and Lunacy arrive at the same moment at a festival to which Jupiter has convened all the Gods. Lunacy, full of arrogance, wishes to enter the banquet-hall before Love, and in order to do so turns everything topsy-turvy to secure his end. The vindictive Love, in order to be avenged, discharges a flight of arrows from the historical quiver; but Lunacy avoids these by becoming invisible, and in his wrath pulls out Love's eyes, but afterwards skilfully puts them back in place with a bandage.

Love, in despair at being blinded, goes to implore the help of his mother. The latter desires the boy to remove the bandages from his eyes, but his efforts are useless; they are full of knots. Venus calls on Jupiter for justice for the injury done her boy. The Father of Gods accepts the position of arbitrator and cites the offender to appear before his tribunal. Mercury acts as attorney for Lunacy and Apollo does the special pleading for Love. In the cross-examination, Love tries to inform Jupiter of the fashions of loving, and tells him if he desires true affection and happiness to descend to earth, drop all appearances of greatness, and, under the guise of a simple mortal, seek to captivate some earthly beauty. Apollo, speaking for his client, young Cupid, is so eloquent that all the assemblage of Gods is seduced by his oratory, and condemns Lunacy without even giving him a hearing. But Jupiter is impartial in his tribunal, and allows Mercury to argue for the defense. The latter pleads, in turn, with such eloquence that one-half the jury is ready to say that Lunacy is not guilty—at least among Olympian jurors. Jupiter is undecided; he is very wise, however, and makes the following decision. "Owing to the differences of witnesses and the importance of the case, we have set the case for a re-hearing in three times seven times nine centuries—18,900 years—until which time Folly, or Lunacy, shall lead the Blind (Cupid) anywhere she chooses to go; and, at the end of the time named, should Cupid's eyes be restored, the Fates may decree otherwise."

Lunacy and Love are thus rendered inseparable and eternal on earth; they are connected together for the happiness of humanity and the delight of psychologists, philosophers and moralists, who will always find in these subjects something new for meditation and study. Need we add, also, that the alienists will secure any number of clients owing to Jupiter's decision?

Let us now turn to a brief mention of

THE TREASURER'S WIFE.

This comedy, by Jacques Grevin, a medical poet, born at Clermont, was written in the sixteenth century. This physician, from his earliest youth, was enamored with the daughter of one of his confreres, Charles Etienne; she was a noted beauty, but preferred another doctor, Jean Liebaut, the author of "La Maison Rustique," to our poet. In order to console himself for the loss of his sweetheart, Grevin commenced to write rhymes, and even surpassed Jodelle, the author of "Cleopatra and Dido," by his fecundity. He followed Marguerite de France, wife of the Duke of Savoy, to whom he was family physician, to Turin, and died there in 1570.

He left several plays in verse, the principal one of which was "La Tresoriere," an adulterous comedy relating to the intrigue of a financier's wife. It is only of medical interest inasmuch as it alludes to syphilis, which at the time this play was written prevailed in Europe almost as an epidemic, and as a study of the morals of the epoch is not without interest to the syphilographer. The author, probably owing to his early disappointment in love, had but a poor opinion of the virtue of the women in his century, and makes many odd comparisons, as, for instance:

"Woman, 'tis often been said,

Resembles a church lamp bright,

That hangs on the altar overhead,

And outshines the candles at night;

She sheds an equal light on all,

But without her light, no shadows fall."

He was no believer in the morality of the aristocratic classes, and alludes to the laxity of social rules and the spread of syphilis in the following lines:

"Aussi la femme a beau changer

Un familier a l'etranger,

L'etranger au premier venu,

Toujours son cas est maintenu

En son entier, si d'aventure

Elle n'y mele quelqu' ordure."

The reference to the syphilis is here found in the two last lines; if she has a love affair, there is ordure in the result. The allusion in other passages is much more apparent, but too impolite for an English rendering.

Let us now turn to another curious old French play,

LUCILLE AND INNOCENCE UNCOVERED.

Pharmacists, even at the present day, notwithstanding the rigid laws to the contrary, often sell narcotics without a prescription. That the modern druggist only follows the custom of his ancestor is evidenced by this comedy of the sixteenth century, by Louis Le Jars, *i.e.*, "Lucille."

The plot is as follows: At the moment a rich banker gives the hand of his daughter Lucille to the Baron Saint Amour, he learns that the former has been already secretly married to one of his clerks, a young man named Ascagne. In his wrath the banker places a pistol at Ascagne's head, offering him at the same moment a goblet of poison, giving him his choice as to the manner of death. Ascagne chooses poison, and bravely drinks half the goblet and falls down, apparently inanimate. The father then has the body of Ascagne carried into his daughter's presence, and also the remaining half-goblet of poison; the young woman does not hesitate to drain the other half of the poison to the dregs, and drops to the floor, like Ascagne, without consciousness.

Almost immediately following this double poisoning, a courier arrives and demands Ascagne, who turns out to be the son of the King of Poland. The banker is in despair, and sends post-haste for the apothecary who furnished the poison, and the druggist forthwith declare that the mixture is only a narcotic, the effects of which he can soon neutralize. Scene of overpowering tenderness and joy, and marriage over again to a real Prince.

It sometimes happens that physicians themselves give away opiates without regard for the rights of the *medicamentarius renenum coquens* of the neighborhood. Jean Auvray, Member of the French Parliament and poet, evidences this fact in a tragio-comedy entitled "Innocence Uncovered." This little play is only a rural version of Phedra and Hippolyte. Marsilie, in fact, is in love with Fabrice, the son of Phocus, her husband, by a former marriage. Her passion for the young man is so violent that she falls ill, and in a visit made her by Fabrice the latter learns of the love his step-mother bears him, but loyally repulses her advances. Marsilie, reflecting on the infamy of her conduct, wishes to kill herself in a fit of remorse; but to prevent this and calm her, Fabrice promises that if she will not suicide he will visit her when his father is absent from home. Phocus soon starts on a journey. Marsilie recalls to Fabrice the promise he made, but Fabrice answers her offers with contempt and quits her presence overcome with horror. Acting under the advice of her maid servant, through fear that the young man may tell his father of her perfidy, Marsilie consents to poison Fabrice, and sends her *valet*, Thomas, to see a doctor and thus secure poison. The unfortunate *valet* is very much embarrassed and cannot tell the physician exactly what he desires, and in order to obtain some deadly drug he details the symptoms of an imaginary malady, and descants in the following manner: "Sir, for several days past my master, who exceeds the Persians as a gourmand in the cooking of delicious meats, gave a grand dinner party, equal to that of the Gods at the wedding festival of Thetis. Now, know that I, his principal servant, sat behind him; there by his order I tasted every dish brought in by the butler, when such a terrible fury broke forth in my belly that I was overcome with fright and agony. The rumblings and grumblings in my interior were only comparable to the reverberation of thunder claps among the highest crags of Tartarus. Hell was astonished and our castle walls shook," etc., etc.

This narration, which is made in French rhyme and is too long for reproduction, naturally leads the doctor to prescribe for the impudent *valet*, who proposes to pay him a hundred crowns for enough poison to kill his master. The physician is angry and revengeful at the same time at the *valet's* dreadful proposition, but, restraining himself, he accepts the gold and gives Thomas in place of poison only a soporific liquor; this the valet brings to his mistress, Marsilie. Now, Antoine, the only son of Marsilie by Phocus, returning from the chase, sees the flagon of liquor, and, mistaking it for wine, swallows the contents at one draught. He falls to the floor unconscious and all believe him dead. Marsilie accuses Fabrice of poisoning his stepbrother;

the unfortunate young man is taken before the judge, who condemns him to death; he is about to be executed, when the physician enters on the scene, tells all that has passed, and restores to life the supposed dead Antoine.

Marsilie is tried and found guilty and repudiated by her husband and family; and Fabrice becomes dearer than ever to his father. Without making further commentaries on this piece, we see the place occupied on the stage by medicine in the Middle Ages and the social standing of the physician in polite society. We also note the *irregular* practice of the doctor, as well as the high standard of professional honor he maintained in many instances.

THE GOUT.

This tragedy, in poetic form, was composed towards the close of the sixteenth century by J. D. L. Blambeausaut. It has only three scenes, and depicts the triumph of the gout. The poet describes an old man overcome by the multiple pains of podagra, praying to obtain some slight respite from the atrocious and agonizing pain he endures. The Gout, an ever malevolent deity, rejects the old man's prayer for help, but carries him into a gathering of doctors who are vaunting, in mutual admiration society fashion, their power in jugulating all forms of disease and exalting their specifics for every known affection. In order to punish these arrogant disciples of Æsculapius for their presumption, the Gout gives them all the disease that bears his name, and afterwards jeers at their impotent efforts to cure themselves of aching joints.

This tragedy, name given by the author of the poem, is a very curious treatise on the gout in rhyme, in which we find all the pathogenetic theories given credence before the time that medical chemistry revealed the action of an excess of uric acid in the organism. The blood, bile, peccant humors settling in the parts affected were, as we all know, causes attributed to diathesis by the majority of medical authors of the Middle Ages. Thus the gout-afflicted man, in his imprecations against what he calls "the torturer of humanity," comes to say:

"From the top of my head to the end of my toes

I am cruelly tortured by agony's woes,

Filled up with black blood and billious humor,

My flesh seems to pulsate like a sore tumor.

The eating and gnawing I can't describe well;

My tendons all ache with the twinges of Hell,

While through my fingers pains cut like a knife

And add to my torment! I'm weary of life."

Meantime our patient does not appear to have a robust faith in the humoral theories of his physician, for he adds, in accursing the malady that has ruined his health, that it permits him no repose:

"Mal que jamais l'homme n'a pu comprendre

Qui le plus sage induirait a se pendre."

That is to say, that the doctors do not understand how to manage the disease, a common idea among patients who are not cured of their malady as speedily as they desire.

In one of the scenes the gout addresses a pompous eulogy on its power over humanity, and inveighs against those physicians who discover a new specific against gout every day. This list of remedies for the disease is appalling; we cull but a few to satisfy the reader's curiosity:

"One advises flea wort and a parsley pill,

One eats fruit at morning, when with gout he's ill,

One chews leaves of lettuce, one takes wild purslain;

Another smells pond lilies, when he doth complain.

Some remedies most curious are for gout deemed good,

Such are herbs and simples to purify the blood;

Angelica and gentian, the iris and green thyme,

Along with fresh culled myrtle will cure it all the time;

Hyssop and lavender, cherry and water cress,

Basil, hops and anise, all make the pain grow less.

Lentills, sage and savory, when the bowels they unbind,

And the marvelous merchoracan that comes from far off Ind.

There's the beauteous laurel leaf that crowneth bard and king,

Privet and cardamoms, whose praise we often sing.

And there's the sleeping poppy, what peace within it resides,

Culled by the Turkish houris in the garden Hesperides;

There's the soothing comfrey and the glorious hoarhound,

And the magic betal nut, in tropic isles that's found;

There's the fragrant *fleur de lis*, when with pain you cry,

There's the odorous sheep dung, given always on the sly.
Some dote on peach blossoms; some on saffron red,
Some like hyoscyamus mixed with piss-a-bed;
There's bread crumbs and fennel mixed with young carrots
Pounded in a mortar along with eschalots.
There are some who use an ointment this disease to heal,
Made of rinds of citron and golden orange peel,
With frankencense and veratria root, to ease gouty pain,
Applied to the great toes on the leaves of green plantain.
There's saltpeter ointment too, when to the foot applied
It makes the patient furious wroth, or else he's terrified,
Giving the gout new twinges, and the sufferer spasms
Only eased by eggs and flour in a soft cataplasm.
Some patients take a razor and their own flesh deeply cut;
The wound then duly poulticed is with meal and Cyprus nut.
Some take red cabbage when other methods fail
And eat it with vinegar mixed with the slime of snail;
Some use biting dressings made from ugly lizards,
Pounded up with doe's hoof and weasel gizzards.
Many think a certain and most efficacious cure
Is a little blue stone ointment mixed with man's ordure,
And a celebrated surgeon, a knight of great renown,
Used virgin urine as a cure for all the men in town.
Some wear charms like foxes' tails, or a beaver tooth;
Others boil a new born caul and chew it up, forsooth," etc., etc., *ad nauseam*.

Such are a few of the drugs employed against the gout, and certainly we cannot enumerate all the remedies spoken of by this malevolent demon. The treatment of Alexander Trallian, for example, is no less odd than many of the recipes given in this poetic formulary; it was composed of myrrh, coral, cloves, rue, peony and birthwort pounded together and mixed in certain proportions, and prescribed as an antidote to the gout for the space of 365 days, in the following manner: To be taken for 100 consecutive days, and then omitted for thirty days; then taken for another 100 days, with fifteen days omission afterwards; finally, every other day for 360 days. Circumcision was also a remedy, only applicable to Christians for obvious reasons.[98]

This treatment is an example of the methodical system, and "rests upon superstitious gifts," says Sprengel. But there are some merits discoverable even in this apparent superstition, i.e., the great truth that the gout is a constitutional disease produced by luxury, and consequently incurable by medicines; a severe regimen being imposed, at the same time foolish prescriptions were given; it was the dieting and not the formula that made Alexander Trallian's treatment so successful. However, it must not be forgotten that some medicines had a powerful effect in attenuating the violence of the gouty attack; it was for this reason that Cœlius Aurelianus resorted to purgatives and mineral waters; and among the drugs used by chance in the Middle Ages were found the flowers and bulbs of colchicum; the haughty Demon of Gout dared not treat this remedy with disdain.

Meantime the *Gout* addressed the following lines to the physicians and *mires* of the age.

"Gardez vous, Siriens;

Menteurs magiciens,

Vendeurs de theriaque,

Qu'elle ne vous attaque."

To call the doctor of ancient times a "*vender of Theriacum*" was an insult to professional pride. This absurd remedy was invented by one of Nero's slaves, and held a high place in public estimation. "It was laid down in the pharmacopœias, *ad ostentationem artis*," says Pliny, "and enjoyed a reputation that was never justified by its thirty-six ingredients and the varied assortment of inert gums entering into its composition."

In the third scene of the tragedy, the Demon Gout, recalls to the memory of the doctors of the Middle Ages, its illustrious victims of antiquity.

"Priam, disposed to run, had gout;

Achilles was too lame to get about;

Bellerophon's saddle toes complained;

Ædipus had big joints that pained;

Plisthenes on his feet, all swollen stood,

- 145 -

Cursing the gout that coursed with his blood."

How many other of the great have wept with the gout?

Then calling his faithful servitors, Pain, Insomnia, and Indigestion, the Demon Gout bids them plunge his fiery darts into his enemies, to burn them with an unquenchable flame:

"Toy, brule ici par des douleurs nouvelles

Le chef premier, les cuisses et tendons,

Toy, convertis leur nerfs en noir charbons,

Et vous aussi, d'une fureur soudaine,

Froissez leurs mains, rendez leur drogue vaine."

With this superb peroration, he afflicts all good doctors with the gout and rheumatism. Since that day physicians the world over, says our talented author, J. D. L. Blambeausaut, have been the victims of this horrible malady. Let us now turn to the consideration of a curious hygienic play, no less interesting than that of the Gout,

CONDEMNATION OF HIGH LIVING AND PRAISE OF DIET AND SOBRIETY.[99]

This moral play, to which we might give the title of hygienic poetry, appeared in 1507, under the name of its author, Nicolas de la Chesnaye, along with another work, the latter in prose, on the "Government of the Human Body."

Nicolas de la Chesnaye was not only a poet but a doctor. He was a physician of enough importance to be personal friend and medical attendant of Louis XII, at whose instigation the poetical play was written. This work is considered by many French critics to be a classic of its kind; it is a poem dealing with all the curious manners and customs of the time, and treats of morality and the stage. In a prologue Nicole de la Chesnaye informs us how he came to be a poet, or, rather, a writer of verses to be recited on the public stage, in which were embodied the hygienic and dietetic precepts of the epoch, together with the medical doctrines in vogue. Let us cite a few lines from this prologue: "Oh, ye who write or attempt to follow copies of ancient works, ye should strive to omit such phrases as are difficult to be understood by the masses of the people; endeavor then to not exceed in quantity and quality their mental capacity and your own understanding. On such an occasion as this, I, who am ignorant as compared to many among ye, have had the hardihood to compose and put in rhyme this little play of mine upon morality. The intention of this work is to make an exterminating war on gluttony, debauchery, inebriety, and avariciousness, and to praise and extol temperance, virtue, sobriety, and generosity, to the end of improving mankind. So in this work I have given the personages of my play the names of different maladies, as, for example, Apoplexy, Epilepsy, Dropsy, Jaundice, Gout, etc., etc."

The object of the author's play is thus plainly stated at the outset. In the first act we see Dinner, Supper, and Banquet conniving against honest gentlemen by inviting them to feast. Among the plotters are also Good Company, Fried Meats, Gourmandizer, Drink Hearty, and others. In the midst of the festivities rascals fall on the assembled guests and give them deadly blows; these villains are Apoplexy, Gout, Epilepsy, Gravel, and Dropsy. Almost all the guests present are more or less injured, and upon their complaint their assailants are cited to appear before a court held by Judge Experience, while the attorneys for the plaintiffs and defendants are Remedy, Medical Aid, Sobriety, Diet, and Old Pills. The trial, carried on in rhyme, is piquant and amusing, and ends in the conviction of Supper, who is condemned to wear bread and milk handcuffs. Dinner is doomed to a long exile on penalty of being hung should he return. Supper is well pleased with the light sentence. One of the attorneys abuses wine during the course of his argument for plaintiffs, as, for instance:

"Good wine is full of wicked lies,

Good wine a wise man will despise,

Good wine corrupts the blood and tongue,

Good wine has many a fellow hung.[100]

Good wine lascivious men will rue.

Good wine, though red, makes drinkers blue.

Good wine means lost ability,

Good wine means lost docility.

Good wine means jaundiced liver pain.

Good wine means a wild, raving brain.

Good wine means arson, murder, lust,

Good wine means prison chains and rust.

Good wine means broken family ties.

Good wine means woman's tears and sighs.

Good wine makes cowards of the brave.

Good wine digs a good drinker's grave."

He then goes on and gives examples, as, for instance, Alexander the Great killing his foster-brother Clitus at a drinking banquet; he cites the opinions of Saint Jerome and Terrence; he depicts Lot debauching his daughters and Noah exposed to the mockery of his sons; he shows Holofernes decapitated by Judith, and places all these cases to the credit of intemperance. Then he adds a long list of diseases resulting from drink, of which we shall only quote one verse of the original:

"D'ou vient gravelle peu prisie

Y dropsie,

Paralisie,

Ou pleuresie'

Collicque qui les boyaulx touche?

Dont vient jaunisse, ictericie

Appoplexie,

Epilencie,

Et squinancie?

Tout vient de mal garder la bouche."

In quaint old French all the symptoms of alcoholism are perfectly enumerated. It is evident that the epilepsy mentioned by the author is only the epileptiform convulsion noticed in modern cases of chronic drunkenness.

As to the *ictericie*, which a modern critic has translated as meaning *black humor*, it is nothing more than what is now known as cirrhosis of the liver. Nicole de la Chesnaye was a physician; his critical commentator not much of one. We cannot follow this classical author through the innumerable reasons he gives for blaming liquor drinking and his high tributes of praise to the cause of Middle Age temperance, and we cannot quote those original strophes on the ancient satirical poet:

"Le satirique Juvenal

Avoit bien tout cousidere.

Quand il dist qu'il vient tant de mal

De long repas immodere," etc., etc.

In another scene the drunken revelry of the Banqueters is re-enacted, on the return of the convicts from exile, and another temptation to the weak and young and foolish. In fact, one of the youths present, Folly (*Le Fol*), is attacked and badly used up by the villain Gravel. The poor fellow cries:

"Alarme! Je ne puis pisser

La Gravelle me tient aux rains!

Venez ouyr mes piteux plains,

Vous, l'Orfevre et l'Appoticaire."

Then follows a comical scene of suffering, couched in such language as would offend modern ears polite, and, therefore, out of respect to the reader omitted.

In this play are many dialogues between Hippocrates, Galen, Avicenna, and Averrhoes, who discuss medical topics at length, but these are too lengthy for reproduction in this epitomized translation.

The morality of Nicole de la Chesnaye is full of good intentions, but it is questionable whether he accomplished any considerable result in reforming the morals of the Middle Ages; he perhaps fell as short in his aim as modern hygienists on the morality of our own epoch. The same instincts predominate now as in days of antiquity; the society man of to-day is generally a mere digestive tube, serving to keep alive the more or less badly served vital organs.

THE FOLLY OF THE WORLD.

This is a farce by the same Nicole de la Chesnaye. It was acted in 1524, and one of his chief personages in the play depicted a doctor of the period. The following is a short analysis of this really curious piece:

Grandmother Sottie leads to the *World* several persons whom she desires the latter to watch while plying their avocations; the *shoemaker* makes his boots *too tight* always; the *dressmaker's* dresses are ever *too large*; the *priest's* masses are said *too long* or *too short*. This bad showing on the part of the World's workers make his mundane majesty sick. He sends a specimen of his urine to the doctor, who, after a scientific examination, declares the World's brain is affected, and also that his new-found client must be visited in person. On meeting the World he interrogates him as to his health, and asks questions which might serve to make a diagnosis. The World tells the doctor he is no longer afraid of water on the brain, but of being consumed in a deluge of fire. The doctor then utters the following wise and rather satirical observations:

"World! be not troubled in thinking of fire,

Let your mind on that score be at peace.

Know that each monk, and low, rascally *friar*

Sells and buys a good, fat benefice;

Why, even the children, your subjects in arms,

Are born to be *Abbots, Bishops,* and *Priors,*

While church-bells keep ringing false fire alarms.

But, great World, *all the clergy* are liars!

Their flattering's truly their sweetest incense,

Yet the parasites fawn for your treasures;

Ah! church love for war was ever intense,

And their doctrines mar all earthly pleasures."

The World is so impressed by the doctor's remarks that he immediately weds Folly. Ever since, it is needless to remark, the World has enjoyed pleasure without as much dread of fire. It is an easy matter to seize the apologue sought by the author.

Here we see, as early as the sixteenth century, the social reforms begun by medicine and continued up to the eighteenth century. The abbots, priors and other gentry of the Church, who lived in idleness and luxury, holding sinecures for which the masses were taxed; the flatterers of bastard princes, the agents of the rich and aristocratic, ruled the country and made wars costing thousands of lives for the glory of the Church—*i.e., themselves.* These are the parasites that epidemically attack the *World.*

GARGANTUA AND PANTAGRUEL.

Among the famous galaxy of philological stars of the sixteenth century, the men who honored their age, we may enumerate Montaigne, Amyot, Calvin, Marot, Michel de l'Hospital, Etienne Dolet,[101] and the one great genius who eclipsed them all, the immortal Rabelais, who was at once physician, philosopher, politician, philanthropist and *litterateur;* in other words, he illustrated science and letters by his erudition, and merits a place in the ranks of glorious Frenchmen and among the list of benefactors of humanity.

Son of a wine-house keeper, the owner of the "Lamprey Tavern," at Chinon, he took orders in the Church, following the custom of the epoch, because he wished to devote his life to study. During some years he led the life of a monk, and was a close student of Latin and Greek literature; to the latter especially he owes his concise, nervous, but virile style, resembling that of Aristophanes. But soon fatigued with religious hypocrisy, whose victim he refused to become, he left the Cordelier and Benedictine Orders and sought refuge in the charming village of Leguge, that his intimate friend, the Bishop of Maillezais, had placed at his disposal.

Here, Rabelais gave himself up with ardor to the study of belle lettres and science, only meeting socially the freethinkers, with whom he discussed those great philosophic questions that had just commenced to occupy the minds of the really thoughtful. Such superior men as Estissic, Bonaventure Desperriers, Clement Marot, Jean Bouchet, Guillaume, Bude, and Louis Berquin were the friends of Rabelais.

Etienne Dolet, the poet, philosopher and celebrated printer, who laid down his life in opposition to monarchial and religious tyranny, was the very particular friend and adviser of Francois Rabelais, and one day traced for him the programme of a book destined, to his mind, to unveil the vices and console the mass of victims who suffered from social iniquities.

"Yes," responded Rabelais, in answer,[102] "a book truly humane must be addressed to all. The time has arrived when philosophy must leave the clouds and shine like the sun for the entire universe. We must, from this hour, suck from the breast of truth for the ignorant and learned. I will see what is in me, and write a book of philosophy, which shall instruct, console and amuse the brave vintners of Deviniere and the jolly wine-drinkers of Chinon, as well as the learned. So well shall this be done that Princes, Kings, Emperors and paupers may drink gayly at one table together. The *truth*, no matter how hard to reach, and rugged though its nature, must be related as truly as that found in God's book; and it shall be presented in a living form, so human and natural that it will be accepted by all the world, and awaken in the soul of mankind a common thought. What use is there, unless supported on eternal conscience, to recount to good and true men the histories that they love to have related, histories they themselves have made? For instance, the 'History of Giants,' so much printed in our age, since the divine art of bookmaking seems so well adapted to an end. Through all of France I hear told the dreadful prowess of the enormous giant Gargantua; it is necessary to lay violent hands on this history, include in it all the world, and hand it back thus *newly created* to the good people who invented the tale. Here is the true secret; we derive from the humble class of citizens their plain and simple ideas, and give them back ornamented with all the good things that the study of philosophy brings us. The rustic thoughts of the villager, such is the point I wish to attain, in divulging treasures hidden in secret up to the present time by the enemies of light." Such was the plot conceived by the immortal Rabelais, which soon served as a basis for "Gargantua and Pantagruel." Thus, under the familiar form of an impossible and exaggerated fictitious history, following the advice of Dolet, our author proposed to attack in his book all the hypocritical prejudices, superannuated ideas, together with the political and religious superstitions of the Middle Ages;[103] he thus paved a way for a Revolution, that must some day be accomplished in social morals, to the profit of science and reason. In order to change the control of orthodox and monarchial guardians, it was necessary to resort to stratagems, to dissimulate in his plans of attack and use the ideas and language of the superior classes. He had often heard the aristocracy use vulgar and obscene expressions, and he was to put these back in the mouths of his characters, so as to depict their unrestrained passions, intrigues, *amours*, the luxury of their dress, their penchant for disputation, their tendency to sensuality; all these were to be part of his projected romance, which was not to be understood as irony even in the sense of its paraboles.

The official sanction to publication was to be obtained by making the authorities believe that the author was only a gay and witty philosopher, a prince of good fellows whose doctrines were not dangerous to the continuance of the nobility and the prerogatives of the aristocracy; whose ideas presented nothing subversive, neither as to the secular power nor to sacerdotal domination. Meantime, the Sorbonnists, whom Rabelais had the impudence to rail at, doubted perhaps the position reserved for them in such a satire, as for several years previous they had been secretly hostile to him, which was a serious matter, considering their influence.

The condemnation to the stake of Louis Berquin, as a propagator of reform ideas; the pursuit of Desperriers, accused of Atheism; and the red danger-signals waving on every hand, determined Rabelais, before publishing his work, to quit Touraine and to go to Montpellier, where he demanded protection of the Faculty. His natural pronounced taste for the natural sciences, the avidity with which he continually extended the circle of his knowledge, and, above all, the liberty of University life, had long before attracted the former monk towards the study of medicine.

It was under these conditions that Rabelais left Longey to go to Montpellier, where his reputation for erudition, keen wit and most perfect good nature had long before preceded him.

The reading of all the classical Greek authors, and principally Aristotle, had initiated him in the natural sciences to that extent that he was ready to receive his degree of "Bachelor in Medicine" shortly after his arrival at the University, under the following circumstances: He had followed the crowd of students who read theses in the public halls, and thus mingled with the auditors at the meeting; the discussion was on the subject of botany. The arguments of the orators appeared so weak to Rabelais that he soon manifested signs of impatience by a very sarcastic remark that drew the attention of the Dean to the newcomer. He was invited to enter the enclosure reserved for doctors who debated, but excused himself on the grounds that his opinions would not be proper to enunciate before such a gathering of *savants*, and that he was, besides, only a Bachelor; but, being pressed by the crowd, who seemed pleased by his appearance and manner, he treated the question under discussion in such a masterly manner, and with an eloquence so unequalled, that rounds of applause greeted him on every side; his knowledge of the subject seemed unbounded. The Faculty was so pleased that he was immediately honored with the Baccalaureat. This was in November, 1530.

Rabelais had not taken his doctor's bonnet when his great medical talent was fully known and appreciated by the professors of the Medical Department of Montpellier, where his winning grace, good humor, and communicative gayety made him friends everywhere.

Two of his boon companions at the University were Antoine Saporta, who afterwards became Dean of the Faculty, and Guillaume Rondelet; with these men he inaugurated at Montpellier theatrical representations with a medical leaning. He wrote some celebrated farces, among others "The Dumb Wife" (*La Femme Mute*), in which he himself assumed a leading *role*—a farce which is related, as to plot, in "Pantagruel," by Panurge, under the title of "History of a Good Husband who Espoused a Dumb Wife." The following is an extract: "Now, the good husband wished that his wife might speak, and, thanks to the skill of a doctor and surgeon, who cut a piece from under the tongue, the woman commenced to talk, and she talked and talked with recovered speech, as though to make up for lost time, until the husband returned to the doctor for a remedy to keep his wife's mouth shut. The physician responded that he had proper remedies for making women speak, but no remedy had ever been discovered to keep a wife's tongue quiet. The only thing he could suggest to the husband was for the latter to become deaf in order not to hear the woman's voice. The old reprobate submitted to an operation in order to be deaf, and, when the physician demanded his fee for professional services, the husband answered that he was too deaf to hear anything." Then the doctor, in order to make the man pay his bill, strove to restore his hearing by forcing drugs down the husband's throat, whereupon both husband and wife fell on the physician and surgeon and so beat both medical men with clubs that they were left for dead. This farce was played at Montpellier by a company of medical students, and enjoyed an immense run of success. It was this farce that helped Moliere out in one of his scenes in his famous play "Medecin malgre lui."

His literary productions, strange to say, did not injure his scientific work meantime. During the time he resided at Montpellier he published a translation of some of the works of Hippocrates and Galen, and also commenced his "Pantagruel," in which medical history may find some valuable documents, for he showed himself to be in every line not only a physician but a philosopher.[104] We will not return to this, as it is too long, and would take an infinity of time to recall his anatomical erudition, and it is needless to say he dissected as well as he wrote. A very just conception of his style is obtained from the description of the combat between Brother John and the soldiers of Pichrocole, who had invaded the Abbey of Seville, a description which is terminated in these droll lines: "Some died without speaking, others spoke without dying; some died in speaking, others spoke in dying."

In all his chapters it is easy to perceive that Rabelais never once forgot he was a physician, and consequently a philanthropist, for could the author of "Pantagruel" be otherwise? He pleased all those who suffered, especially gouty patients, to whom he dedicated a portion of his work. He states, at the beginning of his prologue, to Gargantua, "This is for those who love gayety, for laughter is a proper attribute of man."

It was this same sentiment of humanity which led Rabelais to give disinterested services to syphilitics, that unfortunate class of sick whom the majority of doctors disdained to treat in the sixteenth century. In 1538 he went to Paris and made great efforts to reform the treatment to which such patients were barbarously subjected; the number of such sufferers was great. He works this fact into the description that Epistemon gives of Hell, "where, not counting Pope Sextus, there are five millions of poxed devils, for there is as much pox in one world as in the other." But Rabelais, alas for modern theories, did not fish in the ether with hook and line for microbes, while holding the white hands of Venus.

It was Rabelais, then, who pleaded the cause of these poor poxed patients, attacked by mercury as well as the syphilis, and who exclaims: "How often I have seen them when they were anointed and greased with mercurial ointment; their faces as sharp as a butcher knife and their teeth rattling like the key-board of a broken-down organ or the creaking motion of an old spinnet."

It is evident he employed sweating baths, however, since it is evidently proved by that passage from the redoubtable "Pantagruel's" nativity: "For all sweat is salt, as is evidenced if you but taste your own sweat, or, a better experiment still, try that of pox patients when they are being sweated."

We know, besides, that G. Torella, affirms that "the best methods of curing pox is to make the patient sweat near a stove or hot oven for fifteen consecutive days, while fasting meantime."

Syphilis, as already remarked, was exceedingly common in the sixteenth century, as will be found by referring to the writings of Italian and French specialists of that epoch. Rabelais corroborates this fact, for he frequently alludes to this malady in his works; according to our illustrious author great personages were not exempt from the disease, not even the Pope and the Sacred College of Rome, not even kings and princes, in fact all the nobility, for we read in chapter seventeen of "Pantagruel": "Moreover, Pope Sextus gave me fifteen hundred pounds of rents on his domains for having cured His Holiness of *la bosse chancreuse*, which so much tormented him that he feared to be crippled all his life." Now, a protuberant chancre was nothing but an inguinal bubo, whose suppuration was considered as a favorable symptom of the disease.

Even the good "Pantagruel" did not escape, more than others, the fashionable contagion of his time, for we read: "Pantagruel was taken sick, and his stomach was so disordered that he could neither eat nor drink; and as misfortunes never come singly, he was seized with a clap, which tormented him more than you would think, but his physician succored him well, and by means of drugs, lenitive and diuretic, they caused him to urinate away his misfortune (*pisser son malheur*). And his urine was so hot that since that time it has never grown cold, and there are different places in France where he left his mark, now called the *hot baths*, as, for instance, at Cauterets, Limoux, Dax, Balaruc, Neris, and Bourbon-Lancy."[105]

The chapters of Rabelais' famous book which most evidence his medical knowledge are those discussing the perplexities of Panurge on the question of marriage. Pantagruel has long commented *pro* and *con*, but has not fully made up his mind; he does not demand a solution of the matrimonial problem from Gods, dreams, nor from the oracles of Sibyls. He, however, consents to take council from Herr Trippa, allegorical name bestowed by Rabelais on the German Camilla Agrippa, of Neterheim, a philosopher and physician best known by his books on alchemy, magic, and occult science. This *savant* proposed to unveil our heroes' future destiny by "pyromancy, æromancy, hydromancy, gyromancy"; or, better still, by "necromancy I will make a spirit rise from the dead, like Apollonius of Tyana to Achilles, like the Witch of Endor to Saul, who will tell you all, even as Erichto, dead and rotten in body, rose in spirit and predicted to Pompey the issue of the battle of Pharsalia."[106]

Panurge always refuses, but finishes by taking advice from a priest, physician, lawyer, and philosopher, who elucidate the question. The consultation with the physician Rondibilis, that is to say, the author's friend Guillaume Rondelet, fellow student of Rabelais at the University of Montpellier, is particularly interesting to all doctors by reason of the anatomical and physiological arguments.

The good physician Rondibilis thus responds to Panurge on the question of marriage:

"You say that you feel within yourself the sharp pricking stings of sensuality. I find in our Faculty of Medicine, and we found our opinion on the ideas enunciated by the ancient Platonists, that carnal concupiscence is controlled in five manners.

"*Imprimis*, by wine; for intemperance in wine makes the blood cold, slackens up the cords, dissolves the nerves, dissipates the generative seed, stupefies the senses, perverts muscular movement; which weaknesses are all impediments to the act of generation. Hence it is that Bacchus, God of tipplers, bousers, and drunkards, is always painted beardless and dressed in a woman's habit, like unto a thing effeminate or a eunuch. You know full well the antique proverb, *i.e.*, that Venus is chilled without the society of Ceres and Bacchus."

These reflections on the general effects of alcohol on the nervous system are very just. As to its particular effects on the function of generation, it is admitted by all hygienists that alcohol taken occasionally in excess excites venereal desires, but when taken habitually it weakens the generative functions. Amyot remarks that "*those who drink much wine are slothful in performing the generative act, and their seed are good for nothing, as a rule.*"

Rondibilis told Panurge the truth. Let us now see what other advice he gave his patient, and also note the methods by which he proposed to secure the best possible completion of the conjugal act.

"*Secondly*, the fervency of lust is abated by means of certain drugs and plants, which make the taker cold-blooded towards women; in other words, unfit him for the act of copulation. Such are the water lily, agnus castor, willow twigs, hemp stalks, tamarisk, mandrake, gnat flower, hemlock, and others; the which entering the human body by their elementary virtues and specific properties freeze and destroy the prolific germinal fluid, and obstruct the generative spirit instead of leading it to those passages and conduits designed for its reception by Nature, and, by preventing expulsion, prevent man from undertaking the feat of amorous dalliance."

We will not enter into a discussion of the anaphrodisiac value of the plants mentioned by Rondibilis. We still recognize the soothing properties of *Agnus Castus* and *vitex*, or monk's powder, as it is sometimes called; also that of belladonna, hemlock, digitalis, lupulin, camphor, and hempseed; as for tamarack and willow bark, their virtues are at least doubtful.

But from this passage from Rabelais we must conclude that the therapeutic uses of plants was already well known in the sixteenth century.

Again says Doctor Rondibilis: "Passion or lechery is subdued by hard labor and continual toiling, which makes such a dissolution in the whole body that the blood has neither time nor leisure to spare for seminal resudations or superfluity of the third concoction. Nature particularly reserves itself, deeming it much more necessary to conserve the individual rather than to multiply the human species. Thus the chaste Diana hunted incessantly. Thus the tired and overworked are said to be 'castrated.' We continually see semi-impotency among athletes. In this manner wrote Hippocrates in his great work, '*Liber de Aere, Aqua, et Locis*': 'There is in Scythia a tribe which has been more impotent than eunuchs to venereal desires, because these people live continually on horseback and hard work. To the contrary, idleness, the mother of luxury, begets sexual passion.'"

There is no necessity for long commentaries to demonstrate that manual labor and active physical exercise lessen the natural tendency to erotic ideas. The workingman and peasant are, as all the world knows, less given to the passion of love than the idle and luxurious of the cities. And the reasons given above by the Middle Age physicians are to-day admitted by all physiological writers.

But let us continue the advice of Rondibilis:

"Fervent study diminishes the erotic tendency, for under such conditions there is an incredible resolution of the spirits, so that they never rest from carrying on a generative resolution. When we contemplate the form of a man attentive to his studies we shall see all the arteries of the brain tied down as though with a cord, in order to furnish him spirits sufficient to keep filled the ventricles of common sense, imagination, apprehension, memory, co-ordination," etc.

These rather vague and imperfect physiological explanations are open to discussion, but we all are aware that an excess of work, of intellectual labor applied to science, letters, or arts, is recognized to-day as a cause for weakening of venereal desires and the forerunner of impotency.

Again says Rondibilis: "As to the venereal act, again: I am of the opinion that the desire is subdued by the methods resorted to by the Hermits of Thebaide, who macerate their bodies so as to quell sensuality; this they do twenty-five or thirty times a day, to reduce the rebellion of the flesh."

This is to say that a certain cause of impotence consists in an excess of genital apparatus, no matter of what variety; and we will add what the physician of Montpellier has not mentioned, that this maceration, which was nothing else than masturbation, superinduced spermatorrhœa, the morbid effects of which, on the human economy, are well known.

It is unnecessary to follow our Master Rondibilis in all his dissertations regarding the anatomical and moral imperfections of women, which he attributes to the misleading of Nature's ordinary good sense, which he thinks "molded women more for the delectation of man and the perpetuity of the species rather than to secure perfection in the individual." One thing is certain, that is, that he speaks with much physiological spirit, and that the amiable Panurge is so enchanted with the learned talk of Doctor Rondibilis that he does not forget to pay him a consultation fee, for, says the veracious chronicles, "Approaching him he put in his hand, without saying a word, four *nobles a la rose*, the which Rondibilis accepted gracefully." These coins were made of fine gold, and struck off in 1334 by Edward III., of England. They had on one side the figure of a ship, and on the other a rose, arms of the Houses of York and Lancaster. This consultation was royally paid for in money of the Realm.

If we study Rabelais closely we find he was a contagionist of pronounced type, and believed in no other prophylactic against pestilence except flight from the contaminated country. This is what he makes his character "Pantagruel" do when the latter was in a village "which he found most pleasant to dwell in, had not the plague chased him out." In another passage our author remarks: "The cause of plague is a stinking and infecting exhalation." It must be added, however, that the plague was endemic at this epoch, and people, on the word of prophets, attributed the cause to divine wrath. The roads were crowded with pilgrims going to make vows and prayers at the chapel of Saint Sebastian. How often had Rabelais endeavored to combat these superstitions! As a proof of this let us make another short quotation from the great satirist: "False prophets announce this lie! They thus blaspheme the Just and the Saints of God, whom they make out to be demons of cruelty. These canting hypocrites, the clergy, preach in my native Province that Saint Anthony gives erysipelas, Saint Eutrope gives dropsy, Saint Gildas makes people insane, and Saint Gildus perpetuates the gout. I am amazed that our glorious King allows these impostors to preach such scandalous lies in his realm; and they should be punished rather than those who, by magic or otherwise, may bring the plague into the country. The *plague* only kills the body; but clerical impostors poison human souls."

It required a grand amount of courage to hold and express such opinions in the sixteenth century, in the very face of the butchers of the Inquisition. This courage was not acquired by Rabelais from his philosophic studies nor his religious ideas; it was inspired by scientific convictions, of which the Holy Office dared not demand a retraction, as it did in the case of Galileo. *For the Papacy, from the earliest periods of time, has always avoided controversy with medical science.* And we may recall here the device that Rabelais inscribed in his heart, as on the first page of his books: "*To Doctor Francois Rabelais and to his friends.*"

He was proud of his medical title, and he considered practice (and we mention this fact inasmuch as an ancient writer has claimed he did not belong to our glorious profession) as a sort of magistral and sacerdotal duty, and demanded, as the first condition for making a doctor, that the candidate for the honored medical degree should have *a healthy heart.*

It was for his patients' edification that he composed portions of his books. He wished to calm their senses by revealing to them the great spectacle of the world; and its purpose is all apparent, *i.e.*, to inspire among mankind a love for humanity; having no other personal ambition himself than to play the part of doctor in the *role* of life, to dress the wounds of the unfortunate, to treat diseases of the body and minister to the low-spirited and downhearted.

The strong masculine independence of his character is noted in the manner in which he has attacked all oppressions, be they from science or the Princes of the Church. He refused to blindly submit to the authority of the so-called masters in physics, and reserved the right to freely discuss their doctrines. "Hippocrates, Galen and Aristotle," he remarks, "great as they are, never knew all. Science is the work of many successions of generations, and that which makes its grandeur so mysterious is that the more we know the more new problems are presented us for solution. Science, like, Nature, is infinite." This lofty language deeply astounded thinkers, and roused against its author that same servile Pontifical party that prowled and plotted in the gilded antechamber of the aristocratic chateaux-owners of the day; the same variety of creatures we see to-day circulating, Indian file, through the corridors of our academies, faculties and courts. For the new as for the ancient, it is always the same word of the past, *Magister dixit.* That never changes.

While acting as professor at Lyons, Rabelais gave "a course of anatomical lectures, given with so much eloquence," writes Eugene Noel, "as to astonish all listeners; and he showed his audience how man was constructed, like a magnificent and precious piece of architecture, a thing of grace and beauty, so that the people crowded to the lecture-room to hear him. Dolet followed these lectures. One day Rabelais lectured on the cadaver of a man who had been hanged, and he discoursed on his subject with so much grace and warmth, showing so clearly the miracle of our nature, that Dolet, leaving the hall, exclaimed: "Would I were hanged and I should be so could I be the occasion of so divine a discourse!" Some passages of this celebrated lecture may be found embodied in "Pantagruel;" for we see that he taught, outside the grandeur of creation, respect for life and *what a sacred thing blood is.*

Says Rabelais: "A single labor pain of this world is to manufacture blood continually. In this work each member has its proper office. Nutrition is furnished by the whole of nature; it is the bread, it is wine—these are the aliments of all species. In order to find and prepare this material, the hands of mankind work, the feet climb and bear the machinery, the eyes lead us, the tongue tastes for us, the teeth masticate our food, while the stomach receives and digests." Here our anatomist dwells somewhat at length on the formation of the blood and the part played in digestion by our organs, adding:

"What joy among these dispensing officers of the body when, after their complex work and hard labor, they see this stream of red gold. Each limb separates and opens to assimilate or purify anew this treasure, *the blood*. The heart, with its musical diastole and systole, subtilizes it so that, met at the ventricle, it is perfection; then, by the veins, it returns from all the limbs. The harmony of Heaven is no greater than that of the body of man. One is overwhelmed and lost when endeavoring to penetrate the depths of this wonderful microcosm. Believe me, there is therein something divine; ah! this *little world* is so good that, this alimentation achieved, *it thinks already for those who are not yet born*."

This extract from Rabelais serves to repel the accusation of scepticism so often made against him, and we see two men in the personality of the celebrated writer of the sixteenth century: the *savant* who enriched *belle lettres*, and the popular philosopher who addressed himself to the disinherited of fortune and science. It was for the latter that he claimed from secular power the right to the material satisfactions of life, aside from the opinion of Pope and Church. Rabelais was the very incarnation of philanthrophy and in this above all other things he has honored the medical profession, of which he is an immortal member.

Rabelais it was who wished to be Architriclinus for the poor, for the indigent, the joyous heart of the Pantagruelist. It was to the latter that he remarked: "Drink merry friends, eternally, drink like hungry fishes. I shall, be your cup-bearer and host; I shall attend to your thirst, and never fear that the wine will fall short as at the wedding in Cana. As much as you draw from the tap, as much more will I astonish you at the bung; so that the wine cask shall never be empty; source of all life's enjoyment, perpetual spring of happiness."

The recollection of his youth, so calm and joyous in his father's saloon, "the Lamprey Tavern," amid the brave drinkers and gay wits, with full goblets of the rich Septembral vintage, pure, sparkling, rosy, grape juice, the glorious wine of his native Province, had much influence on the ideas and opinions of the philosopher. He heard again, as in the echos of memory, the merry songs of the grape gatherers, and the Bacchic chants died away in musical notes adown the aisles of the Temple of Time. He was happy in knowing himself to be Francois Rabelais, doctor in medicine, but looking backwards, he felt the vague and indefinable sentiment of poetry, that is ever associated with great genius. It was then he cried:

"O bouteille!

Pleine tout

Des mysteres,

D'un oreille

Je t'ecoute."

Yet his heart was never sad, nor even tinged with melancholy. He dreamed of the golden age of a universal fraternity among mankind and eternal joy, the duration of the soul's exile on earth.

To the Burgundy wine of France we owe this moral analgesia, which chases away passions and all cares engendered by stupid worldly ambition. He preferred the face of a jolly drunkard to the head of a tyrannical Cæsar. He loved the wine bibber's nose, as he says "that musical bugle richly inlaid with colors of gorgeous design, purple, with crimson bands, enameled with jewel-like pimples, embroidered with veins of heavenly blue. Such a nose has the good priest Panzoult, and Piedbois, physician at Angers."

Rabelais did not ignore the fact that these "good drinkers" once had the gout, for he did not forget to give a medical prognosis in the case of the voracious Gargantura. "All his life he will be subject to gravel." But what difference is it though he had gravel, and the red nose, that glorious work of Bacchus? He derived his warmest consolation from the thought that a little good wine heated his blood and soothed the bitterness of life, making him forget the injustice of some, and the ingratitude of others; a veritable *nepenthe* for his miseries, cares and apprehensions. Every good drinker is a sage. Horace had said so, and Rabelais who had read this master of Latin poetry, inscribed on the front of his dwelling place

"HIC BIBITUR."

"Within this place they drink wine, that delicious, precious, celestial, joyous, God-given, nectar and liquor."

But, at the bottom of Master Francois Rabelais' cask was a flavor not fancied by all the world, the taste of free thought, opposition to all tyranny, a Homeric spirit with a sonorous voice whose echo will resound into future ages. Our authors, including historians, philosophers and poets, revere his memory; and one of their greatest minds has said: "Rabelais was a Gaul, and what is Gallic is Grecian, for Rabelais is the formidable masque of antique comedy detached from the Greek proscenium, bronze turned into living

flesh, a human face full of laughter, making us merry and laughing with us."
A similar judgment is pronounced by the author of *Burgraves*, and *Notre Dame de Paris*. Rabelais is immortal in spite of the ecclesiastical detractors who have covertly assailed his memory for several centuries.

A doctor, philosopher, writer, he was the first exception in the positive world, of that profound faith identical with science. It was for that reason that the physicians of the Middle Ages looked up to him as one of their glories; it is for this reason that his works should hereafter be placed among the medical classics and no longer remain neglected by the masses of that profession he honored. In the epitaph he left, he did not forget the doctoral title he always so honorably bore:

"Cordiger et medicus, dein pastor et intus obivi,

Si nomen quæris, te mea Scripta docent."[107]

He did not think in making this verse, that the Parisians would one day engrave his name with his last words on the marble of his statue as witness for future generations that the memory of Rabelais must never be effaced.

[THE END.]

FOOTNOTES

[1] The Mahometans considered dissection of the human cadaver not only as an impious act, but also forbid its practice by their religious dogmas. They believed that the soul, after death, did not suddenly abandon the body, but withdrew itself gradually, until it left the limbs and finally entered the thoracic cavity. Thus the body could not be dissected without suffering. However, osteology was not neglected, and studies were made on the bones gathered in cemeteries.

[2] The romance of Dolopatos or the Seven Sages is the work of a Troubadour of the twelfth century, named Herbers. The origin of this poem seems to date back to Indian literature.

[3] The words are in old French and therefore not easily translated:

"Vous avez oi la novelle

Tandis com li plaie est novelle

Lors pust estre mieux garie

Que lors quant elc est envieillie." etc., etc.

[4] This famous poem, by Perrot de St. Cloof, as a work of imagination, is considered the most remarkable literary monument of the Middle Ages.

[5] The reader of old French can translate the following lines at his leisure:

La pie avoit tel meschief,

Et la Jambe si boursoufflee,

Si vessiee et si enflee

Si pleine de treus et de plaies;

In'il i avoit, ce croi, de naies

Et d'estoupes demi giron,

Boue et venin tout environ,

De toutes parts en saillait fors.

—*Gautier de Conisi.*

[6] In the *Miracles de Saint Louis* we find the history of a cure effected through the royal touch. This cure affords an illustration of how the monks wrote

medicine in the thirteenth century. The disease resulted in this patient from white swelling of the left knee. The following is the veracious chronicle:

"About the year of Our Savior 1174, before the Feast of St. Andre, one Jehan Dugue of the town of Combreus, in the Diocese of Orleans, was attacked by inflammation of the left leg near the knee. Several openings were observable in the flesh, which was soft and rotten above and below the joint."

[7] Bachelor was in other times a title of chivalry or a University degree. The word was derived from the Latin *Bachalarius*. The word was not introduced into France until the sixteenth century. Under the name *bachelor* or *bachelard* were afterwards known all young men in the army studying the profession of arms, or sciences or arts.

[8] See the oath taken by Christian apothecaries and those that fear God, prescribed by the *Procureur General*, Jean de Resson, *Institutions Pharmaceutique*, 1626.

[9] Before modern times medicated baths were not held in favor; the sand and iron baths, so highly extolled by Scribonius and Herodotus, of Rome, were unknown in France. Sulphur baths were recommended in the eleventh century, by Gilbert, of England, in dropsy and other cachectic affections; and by Arnauld de Villeneuve, in cases of stone in the bladder. Mineral water baths did not come into use really until the sixteenth century. Hubert praised the waters of Bourboune in 1570, and Pidoux those of Pougnes in 1584. The waters of Auvergne and the Pyrennees were first described in the seventeenth century, as well as those of Aix and of De Begnols, in Genanden.

[10] Procopius, the Greek historian, born at Cæsarea in the year 500, left behind him numerous works, among which may be enumerated *L'Histoire de son temps*, in eight volumes (*Procopii Cæsariensis Historia sui temporibus*). This history of the times by Procopius gives a full description of the Plague, and is one of the *chef d'oeuvres* of medical literature, one that will never be excelled. In this work nothing being omitted, not even the different clinical forms, it is truly classical.

[11] Georgius Florentius Gregorius, *Historia Francorum*, de 417 591 A.D.

[12] Anglada: *Etude sur les Maladies eteintes et les Maladies Nouvelles.*

[13] *Traduction de Laurent Joubert de Montpellier.*

[14] Black. "Histoire de la Medecine et de la Chirurgie."

[15] The "Chronique de Raoul Glaber," Benedictine of Cluny, covers the period between the year 900 and 1046. It may be found translated in the collection of memoirs on the History of France by Guizot.

[16] "Nouvelle Bibliotheque des Manuscripts."

[17] Satirical writers would not have failed to have spoken of the marks left by small-pox. Such authors as Martial, who frequented the public baths in order to write up the physical infirmities of his fellow-townsmen, to the end of divulging their deformities in biting epigram, would only have been too happy to have mocked the faces of contemporaries marked by the cicatrices of small-pox.

[18] In the year 570, a violent disease, with running of the belly and variola, cruelly afflicted Italy and France.

[19] Gregorii Turonensis, *Opera Omnia*, Liber V.

[20] Latin *corallum*, which signifies heart, lung, intestines, and by extension of meaning, the interior of the body.

"C'est la douleur, c'est la bataille

Qui li detrenche la coraille."

—*Roman de la Rose.*

[21] Sauvel, "Histoire et recherches des antiquites de la Ville de Paris."

[22] In the year 622, Aaron pointed out small-pox for the first time, but it was only in the year 900 that the two Arabian physicians, Rhazes and Avicenna, wrote their works on this malady and determined the clinical forms, giving the prognosis and diagnostic signs and the methods of treatment. Rhazes, physician to the hospital at Bagdad, recommended, on account of the warm climate of his country, cool and refreshing drinks. In the period of lever, he advised copious bleedings, and for children wet cupping. He covered up his patients in warm clothing, had their bodies well rubbed, and gave them a plentiful supply of ice-water to drink. In certain cases, he placed large vessels of hot water, one in front and one behind the patient, in order to facilitate the eruptive process; then the body was anointed before the sweat cooled off. He prescribed lotions for the eyes when the eruption was heavy in the ocular regions. He advised the use of gargles. He opened the pustules, when they maturated, with a golden needle, and absorbed the pus with pledgets of cotton. He gave opium for the diarrhœa and insomnia, and, when the disease declined, used mild purgatives, etc., etc.

[23] Aaron, a contemporary of Paulus d'Aegineta, speaks only briefly of the malady in his works. Rhazes mentions measles in his works, giving a clear account of its diagnosis and treatment. He says that when the patient experiences great anxiety and falls into a syncope, he should be plunged into a cold bath and then be vigorously rubbed over the skin to the end of

provoking the eruption. Avicenna did not recognize measles, considering it only a billious fever or small pox. Constantine, the African, follows the example of Avicenna and reproduces the opinion of the Arabian School without comments.

[24] Johannis Philipi Ingrassiae. "De tumoribus praeter naturam." Cap. I.

[25] Fernelli. "Universa Medico."

[26] "Brief recit et succinte narration de la navigation faicte en ysles de Canada." Paris, 1545.

[27] Gregory of Tours says that in Paris they had a place of refuge, where they cleaned their bodies and dressed their sores.

[28] They designated by the name of *borde, bordeau, bordell, bordette, bourde*, or *bourdeau*, a small house or cabin built on the edge of town; a cabin intended to contain lepers. The word *bordell*, a house of ill-fame, as used even in modern days, takes its origin from *borde*, an asylum for lepers.

[29] Etienne Barbazin, erudite and historian, born in 1696, author of a number of works on the History of France: "Recueil alphabetique de pieces historiques"; "Tableaux et Contes Francais, des XII., XIII., XIV., et XV. centuries"; "The Orders of Chivalry, etc." He also left numerous manuscripts on the origin of the French language. See "Bibliotheque de l'Arsenal."

[30] Pierre Andre Mathiole, "De Morbo Gallico."

[31] Note sur la syphilis au XIII. siecle, "Gazette Medicale de Paris."

[32] "Cyrurgia," Magistri Guilielmi de Saliceti, 1476.

[33] Michel Scott: "De procreatione hominis physionomia." Work published in 1477, but written in 1250, for the author was born in 1210.

[34] It was Fracastor who gave venereal diseases the name of syphilis in his poem "Syphilis sive Morbus Gallicus," published at Verona in 1530. According to Ricord, syphilis is derived from the Greek words *sus*, pork, and *philia*, love (love for pork). *Gorre* in the Romanesque language long before had the same signification.

[35] The Provencal text in the original reads as follows: "La reino vol que toudes lous samdes la Baylouno et un barbier deputat des consouls visitoun todos las filios debauchados, que seran au Bourdeou; et si sen trobo qualcuno qu'abia mal vengut de paillardiso, que talos filios sion separados et lougeados a part afin que non las counougoun, por evita lou mal que la jouinesso pourrie prendre."

[36] Astruc: "De Morbis Venereis," chap. viii.

[37] Jean de Gaddesen: "De concubitu cum muliera leprosa, in Rosa Anglica."

[38] "Cyrurgia Guidonis de Cauliaco."

[39] Torella: "De Pudendagra Tractatus."

[40] "The reign of astrology," remarks Sprengle, "led physicians to attribute the affection to the influence of the stars. Saturn who devoured his children, had, following the common expression, produced the pox. It was his conjunction with Mars, in the sign of the Virgin, that gave rise to the epidemic. Or it was the conjunction of Jupiter with Saturn in Scorpio, as in 1484. At other times it was the opposition of these two planets, as was noticed in 1494. Finally, it was the conjunction of Saturn and Mars, as in 1496. ("If it was the combined action of Saturn, Jupiter and Mars in the sign of the Virgin that produced the syphilis, the astrologers might well think that Mercury could destroy the effects of the disease, which would be better than bleeding or purging.") Leonicus attributed the cause of the venereal plague to the general inundations that occurred about that period, *i.e.*, 1493, and afterwards in 1528. Besides, they recognized as a cause of these venereal symptoms a general acridity of the humors and the pre eminence of the four cardinal humors, but more especially of a metastasis of bilious matter from the liver towards the genital organs."

[41] "De Morbo Gallico."

[42] "Antiquites de Paris," Tome III., by Sauval.

[43] "Observations et histoires chirurgiques," 1670, Geneve.

[44] Antoine Lecocq, "De ligno sancto."

[45] The use of mercury, *larga manu*, in frictions was commenced in 1497.

[46] Rabelais himself had attended syphilitic patients at Lyons, and perhaps elsewhere, with more or less success. He says, in fact, in the fifth book of Pantagruel, that among impossible things it is necessary to class a quintessence "warranted to cure the pox, as they say at Rouen." Now, be it known that syphilis of Rouen was of such a bad type that it passed for an incurable malady. From whence the proverb, "For Rouen pox and Paris itch there's no remedy."

[47] "De Rebus Oceanis et de Orbe novo decades."

[48] "Histoire Philosophique et Politique de l'Occulte."

[49] Cœlius Aurelianus: "De Acutis Morbis." Edition Dalechamp, p. 90.

[50] Magic had rank among the sciences of the school of Alexandria 150 years before our era, in a medico-theosophical sect, whose members applied

to cosmogony the doctrine of emanation. These admitted that demons come from the source of eternal light, and that man might become their equal by leading a contemplative life. There were a number of such demons, all phenomena of nature, and particularly all diseases were attributed to demonic power. These demons were incorporeal, and their light surrounded certain bodies in the same manner that the sun gleams in water without being contained therein. (See Sprengel). Let it not be forgotten that the Alexandrian Library, the richest institution of the kind in ancient times, and the Temple of Serapis, in which it was installed, were committed to the flames at the instigation of the monks, by order of their creature, the apathetic Emperor Theodosius.

[51] "De doct. Christ." liber II.

[52] Baluze, "Capitularia regum," capitola 13.

[53] Fleury, "Histoire Ecclesiastique," Tome XVII.

[54] Leloyer, "Des Spectres," Angers, 1588.

[55] See "Psychologie Experimentale," by Dr. Puel; "L'Histoire de l'Occulte," by Felix Fabart; the "Livre des Esprits," by Allan Kardec, and "Fakirisme Moderne," by Dr. Gibier,—many extracts from the latter having been translated and published in the CINCINNATI LANCET-CLINIC in 1887.

[56] Sprengel, work cited, tome iii.

[57] Tetrabiblon, ii. et iv.

[58] Sprengel, tome ii., et Alexander Trallian. Liber ix. et xii.

[59] Arnauld de Villeneuve: "De Phlebotomia."

[60] Bernard Gordon: "Lillium Medicinæ."

[61] J. Fernelli, "Opera Universa Medicina," liber II, chapter 16.

[62] Ambroise Pare, "Oeuvres," ninth edition, Lyons, 1633, p. 780.

[63] Read the works of Jean Wier in the Bibliotheque Diabolique, with the commentaries of Bourneville thereon. These books have for a title "Histoires disputes et discours des illusions et impostures des diables, des magiciens infames, sorcieres et empoisonneurs, des ensorcelez et demoniaques et de la guerizon d'iceux." Two splendidly edited volumes. Delahaye & Co., publishers.

[64] J. Weir: "De præstigiis dæmonum et incantationibus."

[65] Capeifuge.

[66] Monstrellet, *Chroniques*, liber, III.

[67] Jacques Duclerc, *Memoires*, liber IV., cap. IV.

[68] We find proof of this fact in the works of Gautier Coinsi, who wrote on "magicians" as early as 1219, He gave such sorcerers the name *tresgetteres*.

"En la ville une gieve avoit

Qui tant d'engien et d'art savoit

De tresgiet d'informanterie,

De barat et d'enchanterie

Que devant li apartement

Faisoit venir a parlement

Les ennemis et les deables."

[69] Calmeil's work, before cited, p. 103.

[70] "Ecole du pur Amour de Dieu ouverte aux Scavants." Work cited by P. Dufour.

[71] "Lettres au sujet de la magie, des malefices et des Sorciers," Paris, 1725.

[72] Remigius, "Demonolatriæ libritres," Lugd, 1595, p. 55.

[73] Thomas Erastus, "De Lamiis."

[74] Nider: "In malleo maleficorum."

[75] The ecstasy takes a sublime and contemplative character if, during watchfulness, the soul looks upwards to the Divinity; the hallucinations are erotic, on the other hand, if the mind and heart dwell on dreams of love; when the thoughts are obscene during the wakeful period, lascivious sensations are apt to follow. With irritation of the sexual organs, male or female, come illusions, which are mistaken for diabolical practices on the part of demons. (See Esquirol.)

There is considerable of a correlation between chronic metritis and obscene dreams.

[76] Mental suggestions.

[77] F. Willis observed a similar outbreak in 1700 in a convent at Oxford, England, where the barking fit was followed by convulsions and finally pronounced mania.

Reulin and Hecquet described a similar epidemic in 1701, characterized by meowing like cats, which were heard every day at the same hour among a crowd of nuns in a convent of Paris. These nuns all suddenly ceased meowing when they were accused and told if the thing re-occurred they should all be taken out and horse-whipped by a company of soldiers, who were stationed at the convent door to carry out the order. See "Traite des affections vaporeuses."

[78] Mind reading?

[79] "Histoire des Diables," p. 57 et 58.

[80] That is to say, particular states of sensation among certain beings, conditions which may be produced artificially, with the development of lucidity, in proportion to the power of the hypnotizer.

[81] Manuscript in the Bibliotheque Nationale. Published for the first time by M. A. Benet, Paris, 1883.

[82] For full report the reader is referred to the original French.— TRANSLATOR.

[83] Zoellner, "Wissenschaftliche Abhandlungen," 1877 and 1881.

[84] When we question the Fakirs of India as to the phenomena of *Spiritualism*, they answer that they are produced by spirits. "The Spirits" they say are the Souls of our ancestors, serving us now as *mediums*; we loan them our natural fluid to combine with theirs, and by this mixture they establish a *fluid body*, by the aid of which they act on matter, as you have seen." (Paul Gibier, "Le Spiritisme.")

[85] To give an idea of the ignorance of the *materialistic* school of *so-called scientists*, it is only necessary to read the word "Somnambulism" as defined in "Littres Dictionary of Medicine," where we find the following lines on *rappings*: "These sounds are due to a slight previous displacement of the patella, of the tibia on the femur, when the tendon of the long lateral peroneal suddenly brings the parts back to their first position. This displacement is induced by muscular contraction and can be easily cultivated by habit." The author of this definition supports his statement by the *pretended experiments* of Flint and Schiff; he might have said more justly on *the mere assertion* of Jobert de Lamballe and Velpeau, *who have all committed*, as is well known, *in this connection a grave and stupid error in physiology.*"

[86] Mr. and Mrs. L. B. are intimate friends of Dr. Puel, but the the lady, who is a medium, gives us her mediumistic services in a most disinterested manner; besides, she and her husband occupy a social position which places them far beyond the need or desire for pecuniary compensation.

[87] One of my friends, L. B., always has a wax taper in his hand, which he lights from time to time, in order to find whether any fraud is manifest.

[88] Recital of M. Jacolliot, Judge of the Tribunal at Pondichery, India. Cited by Dr. Gibier.

[89] Dr. Gibier, "Le Spiritisme," 1887. In the experiments made by Mr. Oxon, of the University of Oxford, with the mediums Slade and Monck, spontaneous writing was obtained, under the following conditions: The slates were new, marked with a sign, and closely bound together. Oxon never lost sight of these slates and held down his hand on them for the time being. They were never out of his possession after he had washed and marked them. These experiments were made under a full glare of light.

[90] Pierre Le Loyer: Discussions and histories of spectres, visions, apparitions of men, angels, demons, and spirits making themselves visible to men. 1605. Paris, Bibliotheque de l'Arsenal. 1225. S. A., in 4°.

[91] There was at Athens a house which passed as being haunted by a phantom. The philosopher, Athenodorus, rented this mansion. The first night he occupied the same, while engaged in his studies, he heard and saw a spirit, that made repeated signs to him to follow; he accordingly followed this shade of the departed into the courtyard, where the ghost disappeared. Athenodorus marked the spot of ground on which the spirit had last stood, and next day asked the town magistrate to dig up the earth at the place named; there they found bones loaded with chains, which were released and given decent sepulture, with all due funeral honors. The phantom returned no more (Pliny the Younger, Letters VII et XXVII).

This is almost the history of the experience of Kate Fax at Hydesville.

[92] As examples of responses obtained by psychography, we may cite the following definitions given by Eugene Nus and his collaborateurs, artists, philosophers, and men of letters:

Physics.—Knowledge of material forces that produce life and the organism of worlds.

Chemistry.—Study of different properties of materials, either simple or composite.

Mathematics.—Properties of forces and numbers flowing from the universal laws of order.

Electricity.—Direct force from the earth, emanating from particular life to worlds.

Magnetism.—Animal force, holding persons together; bond of universal life.

Galvanism and Electro-Magnetism.—Combined forces of earthly and animal life.

[93] "I am attacked by two classes of different persons," says Galvani, "the *savants* and the ignorant; all torment and ridicule me, calling me *the dancing master of frog legs*. Meantime, I believe I have discovered one of the great forces of Nature."

[94] Laplace; "Traite du calcul des probabilités."

[95] Olivier Basselin was the proprietor of a mill in the valley of Vire, where he composed his little poems; hence, he named his rhymes "Vaux de Vire."

[96] This is, to a certain extent, a dialect poem, and bears a close resemblance in more than one respect to Tennyson's "Northern Farmers".

[97]

"Et mon orine

Vous dit elle que je meure?"

[98]

"On pense estre guari par l'obscure parole

De quelque charlatan qui le pipe et le vole;

Un autre plus niais me fait exorciser,

Ou par un circoncis se fait cabaliser."

[99] In the old French text, "Condampnacion des bancquetz a la louenge de diepte et sobriete pour le prouffit du corps humain."

[100] Poetic license in such rhymes unlimited.

[101] The group of poets of the same period was composed of Ronsard, Du Bellay, Jodelle, Dorat, Belleau, Bail, and last, but not least, Pontus de Thiard.

[102] Eugene Noel, "Rabelais medecin, ecrivain et philosophe."

[103] In the happy Abbey of Theleme, that Gargantua builds, we see the inscription of Fourier's phalanctory destined for the elect, with the inscription over the great door:

"Ci n' entrez pas hypocrites, bigots,

Vieulx matagots, mariteux, boursofles.

"Haires, cagots, caphards, empantouples,

Gueux mitoufles, frapparts escarnifles.

"Ci n' entrez pas, masche faim practiciens,

Clercs, basochiens, mangeurs de populaire,

Officiaulx, scribes et pharisiens,

Juges anciens," etc., etc.

[104] The first edition of "Pantagruel" dates back to 1553, and the year following he was physician at the Lyons Hospital, where he made first, *before* *Vesalius*, anatomical lectures on the human cadaver.

[105] This origin of the French thermal sources is very curious, and certainly ignored by ordinary patients.

[106] Agrippa has defined the *role* of those who deal in magic in his work, "De Vanitate Scientiarum, cap de Magia Naturali." He says: "Magicians are diligent students of nature, and by means of previous preparation often produce marvelous effects, which the vulgar mostly deem miracles, whereas they may only be natural work." Traduction de Louis de Mayerne, Turquet, medecin du roi Henry IV. 1603.

[107] "Monk, Physician, afterwards Clergyman, I descend into the tomb. If thou desire to know mine name, mine works will inform thee."

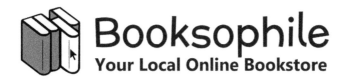

Booksophile
Your Local Online Bookstore

Buy Books Online from
www.Booksophile.com

Explore our collection of books written in various languages and uncommon topics from different parts of the world, including history, art and culture, poems, autobiography and bibliographies, cooking, action & adventure, world war, fiction, science, and law.

Add to your bookshelf or gift to another lover of books - first editions of some of the most celebrated books ever published. From classic literature to bestsellers, you will find many first editions that were presumed to be out-of-print.

Free shipping globally for orders worth US$ 100.00.

Use code "Shop_10" to avail additional 10% on first order.

Visit today
www.booksophile.com

Lightning Source UK Ltd.
Milton Keynes UK
UKHW040911060323
418105UK00005B/578

9 789356 895157